THE SECRET LIVES OF MEN

THE SECRET LIVES OF MEN

TEN KEYS TO UNLOCK THE MYSTERY

JAMES HAWES

ISBN: 978-1-9162790-0-1
Publisher: Hug Publishing

Cover design by Adam Renvoize
Back cover photo by Jo Welch

Book Editing by Kirsten Rees | MakeMeASuccess

CONNECT WITH JAMES

For public speaking, media, latest workshops, weekend intensives and retreats:

jameshawes.org

For therapy enquirers — men, women, couples, teenagers:

synergycounselling.com

synergyinfo@btinternet.com

@oneminuteman1

the secret lives of men

www.linkedin.com/in/james-r-hawes

DISCLAIMER

Names and identifying details have been changed to protect the privacy of individuals. Please note that all of the client stories described are loosely based on real-life encounters. Whilst the issues are very real and some conversations are inspired by real encounters, I have endeavoured to anonymise any identifiable information.

Although the author and publisher have made every effort to ensure that the information in this book was correct at press time, the author and publisher do not assume and hereby disclaim any liability to any party for any loss, damage, or disruption caused by errors or omissions, whether such errors or omissions result from negligence, accident, or any other cause.

This book is not intended as a substitute for the medical advice of your own health care advisor. The reader should regularly consult a doctor in matters relating to his/her health and particularly with respect to any symptoms that may require diagnosis or medical attention.

Every effort has been made to trace copyright holders for the use of material in this book. The publisher apologises for any errors or omissions herein and would be grateful if they were notified of any corrections that should be incorporated in future prints or editions of this book.

For my sons

Cadan and Afton

CONTENTS

INTRODUCTION

THE INSIDE STORIES OF MEN

Men tend to come to therapy when there is a crisis, when they can't avoid it anymore, and when they have been threatened with their last chance to change. In terms of physical health, men are also slow to look after themselves. They will often ignore the pain or concern and only when they have a heart attack (or similar) will finally do something about their lifestyle.

Many men will arrange to come and see me at my practice, but one of the main concerns I have is that about 45% of my male clients come to therapy because their wife, partner, or mum sends them. By reading this book, you're already taking a step forward.

I have spent many years seeking to normalise therapy and trying to find language which would help men access therapeutic support in an easier way. This is one of the reasons I have developed an emotional fitness programme and decided to write this book.

Whether you have chosen to buy or borrow this book yourself or it was gifted to you, the fact that you have made the choice to open it and begin reading is taking action.

'YEAH, BUT I SHOULD BE ABLE TO COPE!'

Behind this small sentence, there is so much unspoken pressure.

What lies behind the 'should'? I often hear this 'should' from boys and men as if they have failed to keep to an unspoken rule about masculinity. Perhaps they mean, 'real men would be able to manage this pressure and because I can't, I don't make the grade'.

When John had entered my therapy room, I sensed immediately that he felt awkward and anxious in what to him was a strange environment. I invited him to sit down and I sat about one metre away from him with the chairs angled at forty-five degrees. There is a small table in-between us with a jug of water, two glasses, and a box of tissues.

John looked unsure and vigilant, scanning the room, checking the exit and taking a quick glance at me before averting his gaze. This is not an uncommon experience for men entering into this unfamiliar space. I am aware of this anxiety and like to name it which often has the effect of relaxing the client. So, I said,

'It's weird isn't it, two men sitting in a room with nothing else to do but talk', I went on, 'I am aware that this is a really unusual space for men, but my job is to make the experience and space as comfortable as possible for you.'

I noticed John relaxing and embracing the space. He became more settled and slowly began to find his voice. During that first assessment session, John describes a series of issues and events that he has been holding onto and has never really processed. He has been unable to talk about them with anyone.

When he first mentions feeling unable to cope, I respond with, 'Sounds like you put yourself under a lot of pressure.'

'Yeah, but I should be able to provide, shouldn't I? I'm not really sure why I am here; my wife thought it would be good for me.'

John tells me about the death of one of his closest friends with almost no emotional expression. In the next sentence, he tells me that he and his partner have been trying to have children for the past two years and how complex and difficult it has become. He feels guilty and confused that it is not working.

I respond by saying, 'It has been really stressful, and sex has become a technical encounter, reducing love-making to just taking up the best positions for conception.'

In the next breath, John tells me about his stressful job.

'I just feel overwhelmed, so many demands on me, I can never get on top of the work and it feels like it consumes me. I'm just so tired.'

John is the main earner in the relationship and feels a real pressure to be the 'provider' and is feeling increasingly anxious that he could lose his job. It's like John has just been stuffing or storing up these incredibly difficult events and situations into himself, not really dealing with them while also telling himself they shouldn't affect him.

I say to him, 'John you seem like you are full up, there is a huge amount of stuff there.'

You would have thought that John had disclosed enough information for one session, but it doesn't end there. John then drops some information into the session from the past. He talks quickly and fluently about his childhood,

'My parents were great, I really couldn't have wished for a better childhood.' —

When clients talk about their parents, the same or similar opening sentences are common, almost as if the inner rule is — Thou shalt not criticise your parents. Indeed, this rule is so strong that it can often block out some traumatic dreadful memories. John tells me how he felt unnoticed and unaccepted by his parents and received little attention.

'They were always so busy, working all the time; I spent most of my childhood with my gran. I often felt lonely and isolated when I was a boy. I didn't really have many friends and got bullied at school.'

John never told his parents about the bullying because he didn't want to upset them or cause them any stress as they were so busy.

Having heard John download this information, I almost felt overwhelmed. However, this has become such a common occurrence for me now that I almost expect it. As you can imagine, it isn't rocket science why John is struggling. He is literally full up. When this happens, men often express this emotion in two main ways. They can feel stuck, numb, passive and emotionally flat-line or they express unprocessed anger towards their partner.

Throughout this book, there will be case studies and examples you may connect with and there are also exercises and actions which will help you work on yourself during and after finishing the book.

HOW TO READ THIS BOOK

This book can obviously be read by starting from the beginning and reading through to the end. However, the book has been split into three distinct parts. Part one describes the complexity of relationships, the relational scripts, and the unspoken expectations men and women often adopt when in relationships.

The second part of the book describes the history of men. This is a whistle-stop tour through the history of masculinity discovering what men have learnt about becoming a man from culture, fathers, media, and peers.

The third and final part of this book will describe the ten keys to understanding men's inner world. This is the central focus of the book. Each part of the book can be read in any order. However, if you wanted to go straight into the ten keys to understanding men in section three, then this part would make sense on its own.

This book details what I consider to be the typical man growing up in a western culture exposed to social and cultural conditioning. My intention here is not to box men into certain stereotypes but to seek to explore their internal world.

It has been written and formulated with the support of research compiled about masculinity and from my professional experience of working with hundreds of boys and men individually and in groups over many years.

Let me clearly emphasise that not all men are how I describe them, but I can safely predict from my experience that the material in this book will apply to 95% of all men at some level. Men are different and I want to say right here, THERE ARE MANY WAYS OF BEING A MAN!

Throughout this book, I will mainly refer to the complexities of heterosexual relationships. The conditioning of men and the outworking of these conditions will also affect homosexual relationships due to the majority of gay men being brought up by heterosexual parents in a heteronormative society.

Men from all walks of life are accessing therapy.

Men are much more likely to access therapy than ever before and about 90% of my clients are male. However, many men do not access therapy — they believe help and support are signs of neediness, or therapy is for 'nutters' or the weak. It is a strange environment; two men sitting in a room, talking about feelings and emotions. I am conscious that it takes courage for my male clients to do this and I respect this.

On my website, I try to normalise therapy by listing the wide variety of professions of the men who come to see me. They include professional footballers, salesmen cage fighters, film cameramen, nightclub owners, politicians, lawyers, doctors, builders, businessmen, CEOs, army veterans, physiotherapists, religious ministers, teachers, youth workers, software engineers, mechanics, consultants, and men from other backgrounds.

I have also worked with men who have been in prison for murder, as well as men who have been sectioned and who have refused to cooperate with psychiatrists and psychologists.

'I JUST WANT TO BE NORMAL'

Shane slumps down in the chair with a look of despair all over his face. He doesn't seem fully present. On his face, he wears his defence and I am aware that I almost feel scared. His body and face say, 'stay away from me, and don't get too close'. When Shane talks, the tone of his voice holds all of his pain, there is an intensity and a pleading nature to it.

During that first session, Shane reasserts his longing to be normal and swings in and out of talking about his life and then suddenly bursting out with, 'What is the point of this, it's not going to help is it?'

I am aware of how difficult this is for Shane and how in attempting to name the truth of his life, he feels vulnerable and wants to look after himself. Sometimes, clients will do this by questioning the usefulness of therapy and the therapist.

"I fucking hate men," Shane said later on in his second session. 'It's almost impossible for me to trust them, to talk to them, and to be near them'.

Shane had been talking about the difficult or non-existent relationship he had with his father and how abusive and shaming he was to him when he was a boy. Shane's anger about this is bubbling just beneath the surface of his life and words.

'I feel angry all the time and just find myself living inside,' he says.

'Sounds like a really lonely and isolating place', I reply.

'It is, I just want to be liked, to be normal and to connect with others, but ultimately I am too scared. What if they reject me, laugh at me and hurt me all over again?'

Shane continues with this shame-filled position.

'Please sort me out, fix me, I've had enough of this awful place.'

Shane was longing for connection and to make contact with others and yet this vulnerability ended up pushing people away. He felt deep shame and self-hate.

'Life is often too much for you to bear and sometimes it would feel better if you could escape this awful situation,' I respond.

'I feel numb, just once it would be nice to feel joy and lightness but all I get is heaviness.'

Shane describes his relationship with his dad and his lack of connection:

'I felt so disappointed that he never showed any interest in me, not once did he watch me play football. He was always too busy for me and yet I longed for his attention. I just wanted him to play with me, but he got bored if I couldn't kick the ball straight and he just walked off or he would only play if he could win, so he wouldn't attempt games with me when I got older and better. Now, as I try and make contact with him as an adult, he is still stuck in the boy phase. I feel that I have surpassed him emotionally. He is selfish, just thinking about himself and his life; he couldn't care less about me.'

The hurt pours out of Shane and he gets tearful. Often as a therapist, I don't need to say anything but offer my presence, my attention, my empathy and show him that he matters to me.

'Dad doesn't like me. I remember when I was seven, it was a really painful event. I fell over and hurt myself in front of a group of his friends and he just laughed at me and mocked me.' (Shane is sobbing at this point) 'He showed me no comfort, I felt so alone and shamed.'

As he cries, I seek to remain present with him in his pain and then say, 'It's such a painful memory that it still hurts right now.'

Through his tears, he says, 'Yeah, I can't believe that it still hurts so much. He is such a bastard, he even called me a total failure when I didn't win a race at the school's sports day. I was nine for god's sake!'

I was feeling so angry as I heard this. 'You didn't deserve that Shane, I feel so angry with your dad for treating you like that, how dare he. You must have felt so humiliated.'

He sobs his tears out and replies, 'I did and I still do. It's just not fair, he has fucked me up. I wish I had a real father figure in my life — I don't want a playmate, I want a dad. I want a dad who can be in my world, listen to me and relay his wisdom. I wish I had a father who believed in me and wanted to be with me.'

When Shane was nine, his dad separated from his mum and became even more distant, showing little initiative in wanting to spend time with him or to parent him. This father-distance can leave many boys/men 'locked in' and feeling unable to express themselves emotionally.

Shane through his tears and his honest sharing was beginning to break out of that box, he was beginning to break the dam that had contained his pain for many years. In a later session, Shane was able to say, 'I've never spoken to anyone like this before. I love talking like this and wish that I could talk to others in this way. I have no idea what you have been doing, but it feels like magic.'

Men can spend many years trying to think themselves out of a stuck place. However, the key out of this box is to allow themselves to feel their way out of it

---

You may have spent many years trying to think yourself out of this box and stuck in one place. However, the key out of this box is to *feel* yourself out of it. You may recognise yourself in this list below or perhaps you are still figuring it out.

TOP 10 REASONS MEN START COUNSELLING

1. Relational and family difficulties
2. Anger management
3. Depression, anxiety, and shame
4. Workplace issues including bullying
5. Sex, sexuality, and masculinity issues
6. Loss of confidence and low self-esteem
7. Emotional restriction and numbness
8. Stress (busyness)
9. Substance abuse
10. Trauma and loss

As we will explore throughout this book, the *feeling* route for many men is full of danger and some men become consumed by shame, self-loathing, and rage. The magic is simple but difficult. I would describe the magic as empathy and active listening and being able to stay with the pain of the other. Empathy is the gift.

'APPARENTLY, I AM ANGRY ALL THE TIME. HOW IS THIS GOING TO HELP ME ANYWAY?'

Ian sat down in the chair and immediately said, 'I'm not really sure what I'm doing here, I shouldn't be wasting your time, in fact, everything is fine. I'm only here to keep the missus happy, she thought it would be good for me.'

'It sounds like you are not sure if you want to be here,' I respond.

This is a common opening sentence I hear from men who have hit a crisis. I used the classic therapist response called paraphrasing. It sounds as if I'm repeating what I have just heard and in a way, it is, with the intention of allowing the client to hear what they have said.

Ian continues: 'Don't get me wrong, I need to be here. If I didn't come, she has threatened to throw me out.'

'That sounds a little scary, it's important you are here because you want to save the relationship.'

The client defences are on full alert questioning the therapist, almost like he is saying, 'If I can't help myself, how on earth do you think you are going to help me?' The client is protecting himself due to his pride and self-reliance and is full of suspicion and anxiety about talking to a professional stranger. The client has to take the risk of sharing his secrets but is unsure if the therapist will be able to manage them.

'It's not like I'm angry anyway, ask my friends, they have never seen me angry.'

'But you find yourself here.'

'Well, about twice a year, I suddenly just blow for what seems like no reason at all. It is really affecting my relationship. I don't know what is wrong with me, I've got nothing to be angry about. Everything in my life is great. Compared to most people in the world I really have nothing to complain about. I thought I had it all under control but now all that is shattered. I feel powerless and out of control to do anything to stop this wave of anger. If you had asked me a year ago, my life was perfect, no blips, everything was sweet.'

When Ian said this, it felt like he had little practise in the art of managing things when they go wrong. He had not developed emotional resilience. When things had become difficult, he found himself back in a boy-state saying, 'poor me, it is not fair'. When I hear this kind of response it becomes clear that his 'little inner boy' is feeling very insecure expressing himself through anger, rage tantrums, and projecting his pain on the other.

During our third therapy session, Ian began to talk about his childhood.

'I was always getting into trouble when I was a boy. My parents told me I had to stop bringing trouble to their door. They would often threaten to drop me off at the local children's home. Once they drove me to a nearby borstal (youth offender's prison) and said if I didn't start to behave, they would send me there.'

'That sounds really scary and hurtful.'

'To be honest, I didn't care about their little threats. Dad would often beat me and both parents were verbally abusive towards me. I was the black sheep of the family; I could never do anything right. My sister was the favourite.'

As Ian said this, I could see the hard and resistant shell begin to soften and I could see the hurt inner boy appearing on his face.

'It's almost like their threats didn't hurt you, you were already hurting so much. Little Ian was doing everything he could to look after himself.'

'It was a normal part of my childhood growing up, I often got into trouble at school and when I got home, dad gave me a good thrashing.'

'That sounds awful, but you just had to get used to it and yet it hurt inside so much.'

As I said this, Ian's eyes began to well up and the little unsafe boy trapped deep within started to squeeze himself out in softness and moistness. The tears seemed to represent so many unmet needs and his longing to be looked after and loved.

'I have never cried in front of another man before, what is happening to me?'

During future sessions, Ian really held onto the language of 'little Ian', it struck a chord with him and for many sessions afterwards, we would come back to the pain of the inner boy and how Ian could begin to look after him. Up to this point, Ian had learnt to look after himself by staying in control, developing a hard and tough exterior, hurting others before they hurt him and protecting himself against the pain of further rejection.

We spoke about his physical and emotional scars and wounds and how they still needed to be tended to. The work on the inner boy was crucial as he dominated Ian's adult self and demanded so much of his time. 'Little Ian' still held so many unmet needs.

Ian was changing and after ten sessions it was evident to him and myself that his behaviour was shifting. Ian began to take responsibility for his behaviour, anger, and language. He was feeling good about his new way of being. He was really enjoying this opportunity to talk to me and said:

'Talking to another man like this is a first in my life and feels incredible. I can't believe that I sit here with you for fifty minutes and time just flies. I don't know where it goes, and I can't believe how much I look forward to this time. This has really changed me.'

As our work progressed and Ian became much more emotionally fit and things were changing in his relationships at work and at home. However, his wife struggled to accept that he had changed and couldn't quite trust he wasn't just putting it on.

Ian told me his wife said to him, 'I'm finding it difficult to get used to the new you. You have changed and to be honest I am waiting for the relapse.'

Having lived with Ian for many years and seen his anger, she needed to test this change. Ian could really understand this. On another occasion, when Ian had been practising his emotional fitness, he relayed how his wife almost felt threatened by the change.

'You are stealing my thunder.' His wife felt like he was now acting out of character and questioning the prescribed stereotypical roles. When Ian expressed his emotions or practised empathy, his wife struggled to know what to do with it. Almost as if she was threatened by this change and part of her didn't like it.

For many of the sessions, we were left talking about his wife's experience. Eventually, he convinced her to join him in couple therapy. His wife found this useful and she began to take responsibility for her emotions, language, and behaviour. When this happened, they were in a good place for growth in their relationship and our work came to an end.

STEVE WAS STUCK IN SHAME WHICH ARRESTED HIS PSYCHOLOGICAL DEVELOPMENT

As soon as Steve sat down, I noticed that he was in a vulnerable place and as he began to talk, his eyes welled up with tears.

'Sorry, I don't know what's wrong with me.'

'It's like your sadness is so near the brim, you are full to overflowing.'

I draw his attention to the tissues.

'No thanks.'

Nearly every time I offer men the chance to dry their tears with tissues, they refuse. They usually use their hands or sleeve. It is almost as if using tissues would be a further indicator of weakness.

Steve began to talk about his relationship with his dad or lack of it.

'Dad is just passive and I'm really disappointed in him. He is not enough and has hung me out to dry. He never steps up. He doesn't care!'

Steve struggled to give me any eye contact and looked uncomfortable. The passive part of him doesn't want to upset anyone or rock the boat.

'I like being the boy and don't want to grow up, I don't want the responsibility - I want to be looked after.'

'Growing up just seems too risky,' I reply.

Steve relies on his mum still to do a lot for him even though he doesn't live at home. Steve would often say 'I don't know'. I often reply with, 'I wonder if you do know but it is too difficult to acknowledge what you know. That truth is too scary.'

Steve struggled to work with his shame, with his sense of smallness and impotence. The boy part of him was so strong and comforting and he had become used to this unhealthy comfortability. He had to take the risk, but some clients are unable or not yet ready to do that work, leaving them stuck in the boy-mindset. This was, unfortunately, the case for Steve at this point in his life.

'I FEEL NUMB AND LIKE I'M JUST GOING THROUGH THE MOTIONS.'

Peter is a good-looking, well-dressed man in his early thirties. He is well-presented and appears to be self-assured, confident, and commanding. He began to tell me his story.

'I don't know what is wrong with me. I have everything I ever dreamed of. I have a lovely house, great job, top car, and have had loads of sex with beautiful women, but I'm not happy. I cannot sustain relationships. I have had sex with over two-hundred-and-fifty women, I'm not bragging, it's just this very issue has become a problem. I love the chase, the conquest and the sex. If I do see her again, it does not take long before I'm feeling bored and trapped.'

'You feel unfulfilled by your sex life. Part of you wants more from a relationship but you are not sure what stops you settling,' I reply.

'Sex is like a drug. The chase and conquest consume me and excite me and once I have had the hit of the climax, it is as if I'm coming down. The sex is not the drug, it's the chase and the power that are the drug and the feeling I get once I know she wants me.'

I have worked with several men who present with sexual dysfunction. This could include premature or delayed ejaculation, impotence, and sex addiction. Sex and the rituals around sex have become a coping strategy and a comfort blanket. For Peter, it was the way of him staying emotionally alive in which he was constantly trying to stave off emotionally flat-lining. Part of him felt dead inside and ultimately stuck on a loop. The sex wasn't working. He felt lonely and unfulfilled due to the mystery of the inability to form and sustain a meaningful relationship.

When a client presents with a powerful coping strategy, then I suspect that the key will be in the past. This kind of coping strategy has been part of his life for a long time and it becomes difficult to break. A couple of sessions later, Peter began to talk about his family of origin and significant events in his childhood.

'I want to get into other women literally, but I can't let them in me! I have such a deep desire to be in them'.

'You want to be deeply connected to women, almost like you want to be consumed or immersed in them'.

'Exactly, but I fear letting them see me, know me, or have any control over me'.

'It's like you have created strong walls of protection and letting them into you would risk the possibility of rejection?'

Suddenly, Peter finds himself travelling back to his ten-year-old self. Therapy is exciting like this when a thought, word, or feeling can connect with a past event triggering a similar feeling.

'I can still cry and feel the pain of all those years ago when my girlfriend dumped me, the loss and rejection still haunt me to this day.'

'It was such a painful experience and you don't want to experience pain like that again'.

Peter had begun to access some of the key roots of his present predicament.

'My dad wanted to be my playmate and mum was distant. I had two distant parents.'

'You didn't get enough from your parents. They left you empty in some way.'

'I never felt like they had enough time for me or that I mattered.'

'Sounds like you didn't feel accepted or loved.'

At this point, Peter's eyes began to well up with tears and they flowed down on his cheek, but he was quick to regain control.

For a couple of sessions, the work focussed on his relationship with his mum and we discussed the possibility of him talking to his mum about his childhood experience.

'I eventually plucked up enough courage to talk to Mum about my childhood. It was scary as it felt like I risked being rejected all over again. Unfortunately, Mum was unable to hear me. She became defensive, blaming me for upsetting her and became 'emotional'.'

The above encounter by an adult child with their parent is quite common. So often, parents can be stuck in their inner child and still want to be looked after. Equally, this kind of response can happen when men share their vulnerability with their partners. Some women can't bear to experience vulnerability from their menfolk and become tearful. These tears may indicate discomfort about what they are hearing and experiencing.

However, when these tears arise in the midst of the example above, then the male feels unheard, closed down, it reinforces the old code that his feelings are not important. His feelings should not be expressed because it could lead to upsetting the female and it connects with the old message that boys should not 'upset their mum!'

What the man hears from the women within this exchange is, 'My feelings are more fragile and delicate than yours and I need to be looked after, you don't'. In later sessions, Peter began to explore the comfort of sex and how this coping strategy enabled him to survive but not to thrive. Sex did not help him grow or develop.

'I love sex, I feel connected, safe, loved and enlivened, but that feeling wanes very quickly'.

'It doesn't satisfy your deeper needs,' I ask.

'No, never, it just feels like a drug addict and I regularly need to get my fix'.

'It's almost like it is plastering over a crack and then after a short while the crack reappears'.

'There is a crack, a crack in everything, that's how the light gets in.'[1]

— ***ANTHEM*, LEONARD COHEN**

Successful therapy occurs when the client can have the courage to explore the crack exposed by an unhealthy habit. Peter had never learnt how to self-sooth. When attachment to significant others is poor or distant, then a child lacks emotional comfort. When a child is not given attention or love when he is hurting, he is unable to learn how to soothe himself emotionally.

Peter had a lack of external love and was still looking for unconditional love, still wanting to be soothed. As a small boy, he had learnt how to look after himself in one way through becoming self-reliant and creating an emotional wall of self-protection to prevent the pain of rejection. He created a fortress, emotionally untouchable, and self-reliant resulting in loneliness and numbness. Peter lived by two rules.

1. Stay in control
2. Wait for the perfect one. She will win me over and know what I want. She will have the magic key to open me up.

Peter learnt as a boy that he needed to look after himself and protect his fragile emotions. He would get his needs met to some degree but on his terms, he had to remain in control. Sex had become the comforter, the soother, the dummy, or as they call it in the USA, the pacifier. This sex dummy is thrilling and ecstatic and the self is lost in the physical and human union. When babies grow up, they grow out of needing a pacifier as they learn to self-sooth. Unfortunately, some adults don't and substitute external comforters are used such as eating, substances, sex, cigarettes, and work.

You will notice something about the above stories and encounters with men in the therapy room. Most of their 'stuff' is not about the present but about the past. They are still seeking to work out what they had been given from parents, peers, culture, and media.

In my work with hundreds of men and boys, I began to notice common traits. Men struggled to express themselves emotionally and women struggled to witness and listen to men's emotional vulnerability. The underlying problem didn't lie with men or women but with the lessons they had learnt about what it means to be a man or a woman.

This book began its life when I delivered a talk to women entitled, '10 tips on how to understand men'. My hope was that this talk would help women understand the mixed messages men were receiving about emotional expression.

In the book, 'The will to change — men, masculinity and love', Bell Hooks[2] reached the conclusion that men will not change if we keep on shaming them and emotionally beating them up. Instead of doing this, Hooks argues, that what is needed instead is understanding, empathy, and support. This is not, I must stress, about condoning unhealthy behaviour, but about supporting men to evolve and change.

> 'You cannot solve a problem from the same level of consciousness that created it.'[3]
>
> — ALBERT EINSTEIN

Hooks suggests that women struggle to help men and boys change and to become the men that they secretly desire because they are part of the same discourse as men. Women, inadvertently, perpetuate the problem. The very women who long for their men to change have been brought up with certain expectations of men, including what a man should be like, what a man should be able to do, and how a man should behave.

The key message of this book is, that for fulfilling relationships, ideas of masculinity and femininity will need to be challenged and changed. We need to have the courage to allow women and men to jump out of the stereotypical gender box.

Both men and women are locked into a cultural discourse and have been affected by gender socialisation. Just as men need to change their view and expectations of women, so women will need to adjust their view and expectations of men. Men need the support of women in the process of change and vice versa.

DO WE AS A CULTURE REALLY WANT MEN TO CHANGE?

Men are changing, but it can seem slow. There are strong traditional male forces in society that resist these changes. They just want things to remain how they are or even to go back to how things were before. Gender politics has never been more in the public eye with the #metoo campaign.

The scandals surrounding Harvey Weinstein, Kevin Spacey, and Jimmy Saville have highlighted abuse of male power and male privilege.

Masculine behaviour is being challenged in a way it was not in previous decades. This has left some men feeling insecure about how to behave and has led to a backlash from men who feel confused, blamed, shamed, and restricted. This is the very reason why developing emotional fitness and learning about gender conditioning and cultural scripts is so important in the work of ongoing change.

PART 1

BREAKING THE RELATIONAL CODE

As humans, we are complex which makes relationships incredibly difficult. It is a wonder how couples manage these incredibly intricate connections and stay connected as long as they do. In many ways, relationships are a complete mystery to us. Our family of origin and early experiences are key sources that inform us about the importance of being and staying in a relationship. These experiences may also keep us in unhealthy relational situations.

I want to name some of the messages we unknowingly believe which affect our relationships for good or bad. This is the story of how we have learnt to be together, the messages and codes we have heard, believed, and subconsciously act out. This internal script is so powerful and discrete that many of us never identify it or become aware of it. The code may emerge through messages like;

'I need to make and keep her/him happy'

'It is my job/role to provide financially and their role to be the main caregiver to the children'

'She should always be available for sex'

'He will be strong and be able to protect me'

'She should be a good cook'

'He should be good at DIY'

We will explore some of the roots of these messages and how unspoken expectations have a massive impact on our relationships. For relationships to grow and develop, the code needs to be identified, changed, renegotiated, and sometimes broken.

Time has become one of the most precious commodities in today's culture. Many of the couples who come to see me for help in their relationship are time-poor. Most of them cannot make time for each other and find it almost impossible to arrange regular therapy sessions. Checking and comparing diaries becomes a source of arguments and busy lives are ultimately pushing people apart.

The couples who book therapy sessions with me typically both work and have young children, gym memberships, and other hobbies. It is often not surprising the relationship takes a back seat. It becomes functional, subconsciously relied upon and is generally given minimal input.

Couples come to me wanting a fix and often a quick fix to fit into their busy lives. I know therapy won't work as soon as they start to negotiate their diaries. If they can't make time for relational therapy, then they will not have time to put any energy into mending or rebuilding the relationship. They want it all and cannot let anything drop or give anything up and so the relationship suffers.

Heather and James enter my therapy room for their first appointment. They both look tired and almost separate. As I introduce myself, I notice tears are welling up in Heather's eyes and James gives me a look of desperation silently pleading for help. It feels like they have run out of ideas and are caught on a relational loop. Many couples never identify this functional state and stay in a 'loveless marriage' out of convenience and fear. There are several reasons why couples come to my practice but the top five are highlighted below.

TOP 5 REASONS COUPLES COME TO MY PRACTICE

- Angry exchanges and constant arguments
- Communication issues
- Lack of intimacy
- Adultery and affairs
- Loss of connection

Heather speaks first, 'I'm just so tired of the constant micro-aggressions in our relationship and I don't think James really loves me anymore. He rarely tells me he loves me and never initiates for us to do anything together, yet he always has time to plan to do things with his mates. I ultimately feel lonely in our relationship.'

James responds, 'You always seem on edge and it seems like whatever I do is never good enough. I find it difficult to know what will make you happy. To be honest, I am tired of getting it wrong again and sometimes I just give up trying. Being with my mates is a release for me, it is just so uncomplicated'.

I say, 'It sounds like you are missing each other and that unspoken expectations and longings have been hidden deep as you both look at ways of looking after yourself in what can seem like a hostile situation'.

Heather says, 'That is exactly how it feels,' and James is nodding as I continue.

'It is almost like you have both closed down and built your emotional defensive walls and assumed your survival positions and then your internal sniper takes a shot at the other.'

This opening exchange is very common with the couples I work with. The relationship has shut down due to self-protection. Highlighting the walls and the self-protective nature of the present state of the relationship can begin to open up the communication channels again.

In the next chapter, I will explore how the love in a relationship typically seems to disappear moving from a vibrant sexual and emotional energy state to mere functionality. The second chapter to this part of the book will explore some of the unspoken expectations which are brought into a relationship and can be a major blocker to growth.

CHAPTER 1: HAPPY EVER AFTER

During the honeymoon phase of a relationship, when conquest, closeness, attraction and chemical 'imbalances' are at their peak, the couple can feel 'head over heels' in love and eager to be in each other's company. They are talkative, excited, and happy with a hope that this stage will last forever. Romance is certainly in the air. He is on top of his game, initiating fun experiences. Sex will be on tap. It almost feels addictive. They feel loved, accepted, and experience a surge in their self-esteem.

This kind of experience has jettisoned their self-love to unimaginable heights and it is difficult not to be consumed by it. Many of us want this stage of the relationship to last forever and I sometimes refer to this stage as the 'romance delusion' which I will explore in more detail in a later chapter.

MARMITE MOON

The honeymoon period cannot be sustained forever. The next stage of a relationship brings the lovers back to reality in which the real work of the relationship beings. This 'Marmite-moon' period is when the individuals encounter the other, their differences, and each other's values'.

The hard work of differentiation begins to bite. Suddenly, love is not so sweet all of the time. There are disagreements. There is negotiation. The other one is irritating and annoying. You dislike the way they do something. You may even hate something about them. This may include the way they eat, their hidden habits, tidiness, and verbal responses. How these moments are handled can be the grounding for the next stage of any relationship. This is where relationships are made or broken.

For many women in relationships with men, they may never see the man they experienced during the 'honeymoon' period ever again. When the mate is secured, the 'hit' is no longer required by the romance addict. She or he suffers the painful withdrawal symptoms of falling out of love.

The addict will often then search for another thrill through 'hitting' on a new conquest. It's almost as if the 'courting' or 'conquest' switch is turned off, as if he has said to himself 'my work is done' and the romantic person, who initially tried hard, disappears. The unspoken expectation (which the man may not even be aware of) is that it is the woman's role to look after the social, emotional, and relational work, while the man assumes the role of achieving success.

Instead of being happy together and 'lost in love', the man now reminds himself that his role is to keep her happy through the old traditional goals of providing material things and protecting her. He expects his partner to 'keep him happy' by being a good homemaker and providing regular, exciting sex. The assumption is if each partner can keep their side of the unwritten contract and make each other happy, they will achieve the 'happy ever after' state.

Most couples are, of course, not aware of these stages and the changes in the relationship creep up on them. When the 'always on' sex tap dries up and life becomes increasingly busy with work and children, most relationships enter into functionality. Instead of full focus on each other, the stresses of work and life can consume the couple and before they are aware of what has happened, the couple individually retreat into old survival patterns or coping strategies. Small fractures within the marital bliss disrupt the 'happily ever after' and distance between the couple starts to grow.

Often men and women will then retreat into their gender tribes to receive some soothing from 'like-minded' understanding friends and mates. Typically, there may be some gender bashing and lots of 's/he always...' generalisations. Women will tend to talk about the state of their relationship and receive empathy from female friends.

Men will tend to deal with their feelings by having a good laugh with their mates. Sometimes, they will make derogatory comments about women in general. There is an example of this which the US film critic Kyle Smith has discussed. Smith commented on Martin Scorsese's classic film 'Goodfellas', which focuses on a group of men in Mafia circles in the 1960s and 70s. Smith suggests that women were unable or unlikely to enjoy this film because there was a key difference between male and female friendship. He said:

> *"When the sex and city girls sit around at brunch, they're a tightly knit clique — but their rule is always, be sympathetic and supportive as each describes her problems, usually revolving around the man in her life. As Goodfellas shows us, guys hanging around together don't really talk about the women in their lives, because that's too real. What we'd much rather do than discuss problems and be supportive is to keep the laughs coming — to endlessly bust each other's balls."*[4]

This is a brilliant example of what happens when gender tribes meet and Smith describes this with typical accuracy. It also highlights many issues around how men manage relationships, mental fitness, and masculinity and how this can often prevent growth, change, and awareness. For many couples, the man or woman will share how they feel with gender tribes or friendship groups, but rarely talk to each other.

THE DISAPPEARED

Somewhere during this 'natural' relational distancing, men can emotionally and sometimes physically fade away or even disappear and their partner is left wondering where they have gone. Often men will physically disappear, increasingly spending time with their mates, working longer hours or participating in more sport. Men will do anything to avoid their partner and the awkward conversation.

Emotionally, the man may often retreat into himself and withdraw from the process of relational growth. For relationships to grow and develop we must feed them, identify and remove the 'weeds', and give them the right nutrients to produce 'healthy plants'. Often, we just expect relationships to magically take care of themselves. The woman is often left with a sense of frustration and unresolved dilemmas, which typically sound like this...

'I have no idea what he is thinking!'

'He never talks to me'

'He is always alright and all I get from him is a poker face'

'I don't think he loves me anymore'

'He never shares his feelings with me'

'He is always angry'

'He always wants to spend times with his mates'

While men emotionally disappear, they are busy constructing an alternative view that women are the complex and mysterious gender.

WOMEN ARE A COMPLETE MYSTERY TO ME

Men typically believe that women are a mystery or from a different planet, whereas they may just be seeing life from a different perspective. When men's emotional survival skills begin to fade and cease to work, they may become aware they are actually the ones who are a complete and utter mystery firstly to themselves and secondly to others. Men have learnt to keep their internal world well hidden. Men's complaints about women can often include the following:

> *'She's never happy!'*
>
> *'Women are so complex; a thousand books would be unable to explain their mysteries.'*
>
> *'She is always nagging me.'*
>
> *'The Missus is always complaining she has a headache, or she is too tired.'*

To remain happily ever after the first gush of romance, the loved-up couple will have to undertake some serious internal work alone and together. Growing relationships do not just happen. They take work, they are complex and love becomes a matter of a choice rather than an addiction. If your relationship is not growing, it could be dying. What I mean by this is that relationships take work and we have to put effort into them. If you are serious about growing your relationship, then this book will help.

CHAPTER 2:
UNSPOKEN EXPECTATIONS

When I work with couples, I am clear: relationships are difficult. There are many reasons for this, but the family of origin and the cultural story we grow up with has a massive impact on us and our future relationships.

THERE ARE SIX PEOPLE IN THE MARITAL BED

Your family of origin experience (i.e. your mother, father, siblings, grandparents etc.) has a massive impact on who you are today. It is the place where our identity is formed and that affects everything including values, morals, judgments, characteristics, opinions, bias, and perspective. Some of these things may be healthy but others can hinder personal development and growth.

Neil came to see me to talk about his relationship. He was contemplating leaving his wife of twenty-five years as their relationship had floundered into functionality. Neil was a very successful businessman and was able to provide for all of his family's needs. However, his wife hated his work and resented his success. He received little support or affirmation from her despite his achievements and efforts.

Neil's wife would constantly criticise him for not being very practical around the house. Why was this? Neil could easily afford to pay for tradesmen if needed. Neil's wife was blind to the positives in the relationship and was stuck in the past. She had not psychologically left home and was stuck in the expectations she learnt from her family of origin. She wanted a man with the skills her father had.

Our father and mother (or adult carer) in our formative years are our key models of how men and women should behave. We often carry the things we have learnt as children into adulthood and look for partners with the same characteristics. Often, we carry expectations which are rooted in our relationship with our parents; when our partners don't live up to our expectations, it troubles and confuses us.

Many couples stay together unhappily or with massive compromises. When starting a new relationship, it is important to examine how much influence our fathers and mothers have in our present relationship. In some cases, this may be in a real and physical way.

I have listened to the story of a female partner who won't trust her husband to do DIY and will insist on her father doing this work, creating feelings of shame for her husband and perhaps leading to conflict. Alternatively, for example, the husband may allow his mother to have a massive influence on how his children are brought up, clearly affecting the parental confidence of his wife and again generating relational conflict.

Parents of adult children often psychologically sneak into the marital bed

There are also more subtle ways that the parents of adult children psychologically sneak into the marital bed. This might include values, morals, rituals, and management of emotions. Many of our emotional survival skills are linked to the family of origin and can potentially impact on development and intimacy.

The unwritten and unspoken expectations can impact on many areas of the relationship, including sex, sexuality, intimacy, touch, jobs, and roles around the house. For couples to be successful in their relationships, any hidden assumptions need to be brought into awareness. Couples need to identify if they are expecting their partner to live up to internal expectations passed down from their parents. When the expectations are identified, differentiation and individuation can begin, leading to relational growth.

FINDING MY PRINCE

The 'dream' that some women have of being able to 'find my prince' is deeply rooted. It's in fairy tales and Hollywood films. It is the story of the prince and the princess. He will be tall and handsome. He will be strong, loving and kind. He will make her laugh. He will sweep her off her feet. He will be morally upstanding. He won't pick his nose or fart in bed.

The script for this romantic idea is accompanied by the 'happy ever after' message with the underlying language used in relationships such as 'finding the one' or 'finding my soul mate'. This is idealistic, to put it mildly. It can be very dangerous and unhelpful for relationships. But it persists partly because like all seductive ideas, it is great for business.

In our society, girls are conditioned to absorb the princess story. Shops are packed with pink, frilly princess dresses and similar commodities. 'Pinksticks'[5] is a campaigning group which seeks to question the gendering of colour and the impact of the princess culture on the psyche of girls. However, it is difficult for parents and little girls to resist this strong imprint reinforced by Disney and Hollywood productions.

Several strong messages are subtlety communicated through this conditioning:

1. Hang around long enough, and he will find you

Girls are taught to assume the passive role and to stay at home and to wait for the adventurer to find them. The message is Prince Charming will find you; he is the active one. This puts pressure on men to initiate the relationship. The subtle message girls take from this is that the boy/man is the risk-taker, adventurer, and the brave one. The man will achieve heroic feats to win over or save the princess from danger. The classic story of this is George and The Dragon: George rescues the princess from the dragon, proving his worth by slaying the monster and claiming the girl in the process. The princess in this story is entirely passive and happy to be whisked away on his horse.

But how accurate is this model of the woman being passive and the man being active? In my relationship, it is not true. Generally, my wife is much more of an adventurer and more of a social risk-taker. I am also conscious the power of this old message is decreasing. Dating apps and websites such as Bumble and Match are doing their bit to equalise the dating game. Women are invited to be more proactive in taking the lead and in initiating a relationship. This can only be a positive thing.

2. Always 'put your face on' and dress prettily

The Disney Princesses are beamed into many young girls' worlds from a very early age. They are presented as perfect with unblemished faces, big eyes, long eyelashes, and immaculate hair. They are slender, with elegant limbs and petite waists. This image of beauty is mirrored in countless advertisements on the internet, TV, and in magazines.

There is a huge emphasis on feminine beauty usually captured by images of young, striking women which many other women feel they do not match. This attitude endorses the view that women must 'look their best' at all times and 'put their face on' seeking to remove any perceived blemish. This idea puts huge pressure on women to wear a mask, aided and abetted by a cosmetics industry worth £9.4 billion just in the UK. Alongside this, the fashion and advertising industry play on any image insecurities. The rise of plastic surgery has coincided, roughly speaking, with the rise of the media and with social media. In 2016, Americans spent sixteen billion dollars on plastic surgery.

In contrast, all men have to do is consider which shirt and jeans/ trousers they are going to wear that day. I am constantly amazed at the low standards of dress that many women are prepared to accept in men. While women dress to impress, their male partners may look scruffy in tracksuit bottoms and a t-shirt.

How often have I been to dinner parties where women are dressed really well and have clearly gone to loads of effort, while their male partner turns up in jeans and a t-shirt. The standards are opposing. Women have to constantly be on their guard to not fail the beauty test, often waiting for the judgmental gaze of other women and men about their clothes, hair, or shoes.

3. Women need protecting

Typically, men's bodies are bigger and stronger than women's. The old code emphasised that women are the weaker sex and one of the duties of men will be to protect them. This old male code began in tribal societies where clear definitions of men's and women's roles were enforced within rites of passage where boys were trained to be warriors.

Since then, many societies have taught boys and men that women are fragile, vulnerable, and weak. They learnt that it is their job to look after girls and women and protect them from threat and danger and save them from harm. The cave or the home was the safest place for women. It then became their job to be the housewife looking after the home and children.

Of course, the reality of this in today's world is clearly untrue. Many women are quite capable of protecting themselves and have broken out of the 'housewife' shackles, and now work in traditionally male-dominated industries and even join the army. The old protection story persists. Boys may still live by the code that they shouldn't hit girls or women. Yet the sad fact is that far from protecting women, men are more likely to be the ones who attack them verbally or physically with domestic abuse/violence and sexual abuse on the increase.

Women are the stronger sex

The reverse of this message may actually be true — perhaps, women are the stronger sex and men need protecting from feeling emotionally hurt. The 'women are the weaker sex' narrative is still very present in a more nuanced tone, through the media, and the comments and attitudes of some men. Can this attitude be something to do with emotional expression?

Due to women expressing vulnerable emotions more readily, and men being conditioned to believe that emotional expression was 'weakness', then this may well be the source of this myth. In terms of emotional fitness, this actually means that women are the stronger sex and are generally more developed and have a depth of emotional strength.

I think many men secretly know this. Men are often afraid of the inner power of women. Men will often rely on women and have great expectations of them. They fear the female ability to endure pain, the woman's emotional courage, and their inner strength. This knowledge can be a source of shame for many men, who are trying to prove they can be strong, tough protectors. When a man feels he cannot live up to the 'Prince' ideal, he becomes vigilant to any hint of shaming from his female partner.

4. He will provide for you

It wasn't that long ago that the roles of men and women were clearly divided. The male in the family worked and brought in the money that paid for shelter, food, and clothes. The female was the homemaker and nurturer. This is still the case in some families today, in which women opt to stay at home as their partner may have more earning potential. However, in many families, these divisions are not so clearly defined.

With the rise of women in the workplace, women have more power and a greater stake in the corporate world. This rise has been rapid. It was only a hundred years ago that women were given the vote. In the last fifty years, women have increasingly become important in the workplace. They now have more power and a greater influence in organisations and companies. Women do not need men to provide financially for them, yet little girls may still be shown these models in many homes all over the world. Some women will secretly want to be looked after as modelled by their family of origin.

Many women not only look after themselves but are also the main carers for children, the elderly, and the sick. In many parts of the world, women have several responsibilities: caring for children or other family members, as well as working and doing all the domestic chores. In many cultures, it appears that women are the harder workers.

As I mentioned earlier many of the couples who I work with are often too busy. Janet and Steve came to see me as they were conscious that intimacy within their relationship was lacking. Steve had complained that their sex life had dried up. During the session, Janet complained she had a full-time job but felt she was also expected to do all the cooking, cleaning, washing, and social engagements. She ultimately felt she was looking after Steve in many ways and refused to look after him sexually as well.

Steve felt defensive, 'You know how busy my work is at the moment. I have to work hard, and I think I deserve to spend some time with my mates'.

Janet was angry and ultimately disappointed. 'And you don't think I work hard in my job? You don't think I would like some time to spend with my friends. This is not what I thought we would become; our relationship looks so much like my parents' and it makes me really sad.'

Many relationships become functional when couples fall into patterns of behaviour that appear to work on the surface of things. When behaviour defaults are challenged then psychological intimacy can be given some breathing space. Once Janet shared her truth - it gave Steve and the relationship an opportunity to grow and develop. Intimacy requires risk and the willingness to expose vulnerabilities. In many relationships, couples provide in different ways and often both are financial providers. When this is the case, men will have to do some work on adjusting their view on being a provider.

5. He will complete you

In the film 'Jerry Maguire', there is a scene where the lead male character says to his girlfriend: 'You complete me.' This romantic notion of the other person providing something that is 'missing', is still very much alive. Men and women are often conditioned to believe this.

This saying is commonly heard and yet it is an unhealthy thought. We often hear the language of 'my other half' as if the couple were separated at birth or that the individual has not reached the perfect union of the feminine and masculine. What does this saying tell us about our thinking or our longings? It says that I am not whole within myself or that I am not capable or perhaps that there is a part of me I have yet to discover and the other person is able to be this part.

There is no doubt couples often create an emotional fusion and can lose differentiation and in the process jettison individuation. It is almost saying, I could never be happy if I don't find my other half or 'the one'. Ultimately, this can be a source of great unhappiness and create a huge amount of pressure on 'my other half' to keep me happy. This notion in my experience has created many relational difficulties, unhappiness, and insecurities and often prevents growth individually and in relationships.

BUSTING THE UNSPOKEN EXPECTATIONS AND WORKING TOWARDS BEING HAPPY EVER AFTER

Many of us remain in unsatisfactory relationships due to being stuck in the trap of unspoken expectations and strong cultural conditioning. This duel trap actually keeps us chained in a parent-child relationship. This is where one person adopts a passive childlike stance and the other person in the relationship assumes the parent or active position. The roles may flip according to certain situations.

In some relationships, the roles get stuck and one partner inhabits the parent or child position for the majority of the time creating a power imbalance and unhealthy relationship. For relationships to grow and develop, couples will need to move away from this parent-child flipping and move towards relating as adults. Couples and individuals need to do the painful work of growing up.

GROWING UP EMOTIONALLY IS HARD TO DO

Many relationships are desperate for an internal growth spurt. Growing up is one of the most difficult things for us as humans to do and many of us would prefer to remain in the state of the child. Women typically appear to grow up quicker perhaps helped by biological and societal forces. Women are often the adult in the relationship psychologically while many men have delayed development. This is, of course, not always the case.

If I were the same person or acted the same way at the age of fifty as I did when I was twenty-five then something would be wrong. Physical growth may stop at a certain age but inner growth including emotional and intellectual learning continues. The complexity for couples is that when they don't grow at the same time and in the same way they may end up 'growing apart'. During the life of a relationship, individual internal growth spurts can cause a great deal of disturbance.

Physical growth may stop at a certain age, but inner growth including emotional and intellectual learning continues

---

For instance, when I trained as a psychotherapist I was engaged in a huge amount of emotional reflection, therapy and discovering many new things about myself. I had a massive internal growth spurt and to her credit, my wife was able to stay with me. I think I felt I was finally catching up to where she was internally. However, it was not long after I completed my training that my wife then trained as a psychotherapist as she realised that she also wanted to do some internal stretching.

My work with men is in helping them to become emotionally fit, to help them connect with their vulnerable emotions, to practise expressing their fear, sadness and shame. In doing this, they may cry, show fear, show remorse and generally appear more fragile. This is the difficult but necessary work of men accepting and not suppressing their emotions.

However, men can often be caught in a dilemma between growth and meeting their partner's expectations. Although women often want men to be more emotionally engaged, when men start to share their emotions, they feel that women are closing them down, shaming them, and generally struggling to cope with men expressing themselves in a new and different way.

'I cannot change anyone apart from myself'

If men are not given a safe space in their relationship to express these feelings, they can end up feeling trapped, confused, and constrained. Some women will struggle to accept men's vulnerability. They may even find it frightening. When men express these kinds of feelings, it may shatter women's long-held assumptions as to how men are meant to behave.

If women want to change the men in their life, then they will have to change to allow that growth to take root. Men are quite capable of changing and as you read this book, you will begin to realise that much is stacked against them and often women perpetuate traditional patterns, usually unconsciously. This book will raise your awareness and take you into the secret world of men. If you read it with an open mind and are open to change, it will help you have more fulfilling relationships.

PART 2

THE HISTORY OF MAN

Only by learning the lessons of the past will we be able to understand and change the present

In this part of the book we will explore the history of man, how has man been created, why are men the way they are and can they change? We will explore the road map to men's present condition and situation and the background reasons that hinder men's growth psychologically. If we have any chance of changing the future, then we must learn lessons from the past. There are no short cuts to long-lasting change.

As outlined in Part One, if men are going to change then women, society, and the agendas for relationships will have to change too. Old and unspoken expectations will need to be exposed and challenged.

Change is difficult. Personal change takes time, relational change takes longer, and societal change will take generations. This part of the book will take you back to explore the making of man helping us to understand how men have got to where they are today.

James Hawes

BEING A MAN IS COMPLICATED

Being a man is much more complicated than it was sixty years ago. To fully understand masculinity and words like 'crisis', 'emasculation' or 'toxic', we must take time to reflect on our present situation and seek to learn from the past. When a difficult situation arises in a nation's life, politicians will utter well-meaning words about learning lessons. Yet, what we have learnt is that history repeats itself and the leaders of our nations rarely learn lessons from the past. However, if men are going to grow and develop it is important to understand how they have been shaped by the formation of masculinity and the examples of men in the past.

To explain this, allow me to use a metaphor from the world of tools. I love tools and have been working with tools for over forty years. When I was an apprentice carpenter, my bag of tools consisted of hand tools and when on-site I cut, hit, screwed, and bored holes through the power and skill of my muscles and hands. If you observe a tradesman today, he will have numerous cordless electric tools in many boxes, needing a van to transport the bulky equipment.

Today, the screw is the new nail! Some of the old tools I have in my tool bag would appear like antiques to modern tradesmen. They would dismiss them as ineffective and too slow and yet when I use them, I get a real sense of joy and quiet pleasure from them. Yet, power tools have transformed what I am able to do now.

As an older man, I can still do jobs that would be impossible to do with hand tools. I use this illustration to demonstrate how during the same period, the world of men has changed. Most men have embraced the evolution in tools and yet they have found it much more difficult to accept the evolution in masculinity.

HE JUST WANTS TO BE NORMAL. BUT WAIT… WHAT IS 'NORMAL'?

For many years, I have spent hundreds of hours working with men one-to-one or in group settings. I have realised that one of the key things men want is to feel 'normal' within the male tribe. Men are on a quest to be normal, to fit in, to be one of the lads. Indeed, if I ask men how they feel, one of the most common responses I hear is, 'I want to be normal'.

Men are almost desperate to fit into the male norm and not to stand out. Their response has nothing to do with how they feel and everything to do with how they want to appear, a state that they want to continually inhabit. Men long to belong and to be accepted by their male counterparts.

Men are on a quest to be normal, to fit in, to be one of the lads

---

Men will often arrive in my clinic as their internal 'normal' is beginning to fragment and feel less steady. Often, their behaviour and emotional norm is feeling a little out of control. When the 'abnormal' state begins to persist, it may be expressed through loss of emotional control. This indicates a state of crisis and they start to look for help.

Many men will reach midlife without opening up and sharing what is going on in their internal world. When they have the courage to share this in my presence and notice my response, there is often a sense of relief. They have remained quiet about their inner thoughts for many years, often breeding emotional isolation. They haven't said anything because they feel scared and they feel ashamed. They worry they will be perceived as 'abnormal', 'weird', or 'odd'. Male silence does not allow men to know what a male internal norm is. We will examine this in more detail later in the book.

One of the key aspects of my work with men is helping them to experience 'normalisation'. This sounds like I am conforming to the external male code of 'normal'. However, helping a man to understand what he is experiencing is similar to hundreds of other men I have worked with can immediately create a sense of relief.

When a man reveals something he thinks is shameful, I will show little surprise or shock and remain non-judgmental. I will also inform the client about the typical internal world of men (described within this book) sometimes known as psycho-educational work. This process is ultimately de-shaming. I have seen men physically relax when they realise they are not the only one who experiences these things and that they are more 'normal' than they realised. A smile appears on their faces when they realise I am not judging or shaming them.

Working with a group of men, this moment of realisation can be incredibly powerful. Men listen to their counterparts tell their stories and realise they are often hearing their own internal story. As they are not used to sharing their experience, it is a huge relief to them when they can admit they feel sad or locked in or ashamed. I watch as men cry with a sense of relief and then this vulnerability, honesty and authenticity becomes contagious.

IT'S NOT JUST ME

Knowing that 'It's not just me' for men (and women) is a huge relief. It provides a release from the hiddenness of shame. It allows men to finally begin their own internal work and to progress to a higher level of insight and maturity.

Many men are 'locked in' emotionally; they are literally in fear of verbalising their feelings

Often the start of a man's healing and growth occurs when he is given an opportunity to share his story and to listen to other men's stories. Finally, he can feel accepted, not just for his external presentation, but for who he *really* is. It is at this point that he can feel safe to be 'soft'.

I see evidence of this in the SHOUT programme, an anger awareness programme I started and facilitate. Having delivered this course for many years, I have had the pleasure to be part of one of the most caring, empathic, and open groups I have ever been involved in. SHOUT will regularly include men from different walks of life, including different ethnic and socio-economic backgrounds.

One example of this care has been the acceptance of other men's expression of their sexuality. Part of this ten-week programme includes an exercise in which men can release physical anger; they are invited to hit a tennis racket into a big cushion, within therapeutic conditions.

The exercise can be very vulnerable; it exposes emotions that may have been contained for years. This exercise had a significant impact on a gay man in the group; he became aware that all the men were struggling with similar emotions. Afterwards, he cried and expressed how partly his healing and growth was due to experiencing the incredible warmth, engagement and acceptance he experienced from the other men. It was a significant process for him and contributed to his healing and development. For me, this was a profound and moving experience.

Men have typically avoided any moments of vulnerability. They feel it is 'soft' to do this. For men, to connect with other men on an internal level is in my view incredibly crucial as we live in a society in which the typical man will be emotionally isolated and distant from himself.

CHAPTER 3:
THE MAKING OF BOYS AND MEN

'It's time to get a man in!' is a common refrain arising from households when something practical needs fixing. This job will need a man who is able to understand the problem and have a van full of tools. This very statement implies that women would be unable to sort out the problem.

Are boys born with these skills? Are they born knowing the names of tools and naturally have the ability to know how to use them? This is, of course, ludicrous, little boys don't have these innate abilities. Does this, therefore, mean that boys have been culturally made to acquire these skills or have they been directed and nurtured to learn about tools and guided on how to use them to complete practical tasks?

Being male is a complex business. There are many ways of being a man and yet it appears that there is a dominant discourse or stereotypical way of 'acting male' which seems to apply to a large section of the male population.

In considering what it means to be a man, sexuality will obviously need to be considered. Within my client work, I have worked with many gay men and while this book isn't specifically focussed around the psychology of homosexual men, much of the material in this book will apply to gay men too.

WHAT DOES IT MEAN TO BE A MAN?

This question is constantly being asked on various Internet forums, which demonstrates men's insecurity in relation to their manhood and masculinity. Many are confused and often live in silence and isolation fearing they may not make the grade.

For part of this discussion, I think it is important to investigate the key differences between men and women. The obvious difference is that men and women have different shaped bodies. But beyond the body what are the differences? What is uniquely male and uniquely female? In this chapter, I would like us to consider some myths and some commonly accepted knowledge which may not always appear as factual as it is presented to us.

Differences between men and women and the separation of gender appears to be really important to many in society, almost like these polarities need to be strongly defined and defended at all costs. Some feel that difference can generate security in defining differences between the sexes. I don't concur with that but it generates strong stereotypes. I find it can prevent societal gender conditioning being questioned.

The one difference between men and women is biological

Male and females have different shaped genitalia, different shaped bodies, some different inner body parts, and different amounts of various chemicals.

Women have reproductive abilities and men are normally larger and therefore physically stronger. The difference between men and women is right there. Their body is the first indicator, is recognisable before birth, and is determined by the 'y' chromosome forming a male from the initial female state. The genetic code and testosterone will then play a major part in a boy's physical development and sexuality. There are, of course, complexities to this in terms of chromosome mix where some people feel that they have been born in the wrong gendered body.

Over the centuries, researchers have been keen to look for and seek to prove gender difference. Below I have outlined the four key myths about the difference between boys and girls and how these have contributed to the making of men.

Men are from Mars and women are from Venus

The 'Men are from Mars and Women are from Venus' discourse is basically rooted in essentialism, meaning this is just the way men and women are and is backed by the often-used phrase 'boys will be boys'. Just accept it for what it is and get used to it. The problem with this kind of thinking is that it is just accepting the status quo. It is essentially saying to men: 'You are emotionally deficient, and it is hurting you and others, but hey, just suffer quietly and go back to the cave. Men and women are built for different purposes and it would be best to honour those differences and keep to your strengths'.

The reason this argument is so convincing is that the descriptions of male and female behaviour often appear correct. When we observe male and female behaviour in society women do appear to be better nurturers and listeners and have superior social skills. Men do appear more confident, stronger, and adventurous. Yet this discourse is, in reality, an observation of cultural conditioning and fails to ask deeper questions of how men and women began to behave in these ways.

I think this message is unhelpful to growth and generates dualistic thinking and positions. The fact is that all genders are from Earth and once we accept this and the reasons behind perceived differences, then and only then can we begin to connect at deeper levels. In the context of travelling, when we travel to different countries and encounter different cultures, we notice different traditions and customs.

We have a couple of choices about how we behave in different cultures. Perhaps, we could be critical of the cultural codes, stay aloof from the customs, and seek to adapt the culture to align with our thinking. Or, we could observe and learn from the cultural customs and adapt our behaviour and beliefs in order to become culturally sensitive. In the same way, rather than holding onto to what we are accustomed to as how men or women are, we could seek to understand, learn and adapt our behaviours, to evolve.

Every man needs a cave

A common notion about men is that all men need a cave. Some people suggest that the cave concept is biological history. It's in a man's genes. He is programmed to retreat to a small, dark, womb-like space. We are told that men have been doing this for generations and it is hardwired into them via their ancestors. However, whenever this 'excuse' for men's behaviour is brought into the conversation, I always want to ask:

> *What about the cavewomen, where do they go?*
>
> *Do they go to their cave kitchen or laundrette?*

The concept of the cave is based on one of the earliest rules boys learn: 'Thou shalt rely on thyself' more commonly known as self-reliance. Boys have learnt this rule from messages they have heard about expressing vulnerable emotions and when adult male carers have been emotionally unavailable.

For many men, the cave is a private 'man only space' and may be a shed, a basement, garage, or loft space. It is typically on the margins of the comfortable, warm and civilised main family space. The 'man cave' could be a space to play. It may be filled with boy-like gadgets and games or full of tools where he uses the skills of his hands to create. Both of these uses could indicate a return to something that is lost.

Psychologically, the cave represents a safe isolated space where the man can be with difficult emotions and pull himself together

The typical man, when psychologically wounded, will retreat to his cave to be alone. Why does this happen? The man wants to remove himself from others because he has learnt that it is not safe to share his inner pain in public, for fear of humiliation and shame. He takes his pain into isolation and muses over it. This process usually includes self-berating, beating up, sucking down, regurgitating and at last pulling himself together so he can present himself back into the public domain in control and with his public persona in place.

Although some will claim this is just how men are, this is not a healthy way of dealing with difficult emotions or relational conflict and indicates a lack of emotional fitness. This behaviour is learnt and is often a basic survival skill in managing shame.

Testosterone affects male behaviour

Common wisdom informs us that 'boys are naturally aggressive' due to testosterone. But is this really the case? I suspect it is a myth for one simple reason, most boys and men do not act aggressively. It is true, however, that for some boys and men with higher levels of testosterone or at certain developmental stages, it can affect sexual drive, libido and aggressive outbursts.

There is no doubt that testosterone has a powerful impact on physical development. Foetal development and sexual differentiation rely on levels of testosterone which will affect body shape and define the foetus as male. Numerous experiments have been carried out to clarify if 'sex chemicals' affect behaviour but the results appear inconclusive.

The BBC programme in 2018 entitled, 'No more boys and girls — can our kids go gender free?' attempted to challenge gender stereotypes. The programme argued that boys and girls are conditioned from a very early age. One experiment on the programme was to dress babies in clothes that were not gender-specific, so the girls wore blue shorts, and the boys wore dresses.

Adult strangers were introduced to the babies and asked to play with them. All the adults who played with girls dressed as boys were more physical with them and steered them towards typical male toys. Adults playing with the boys dressed as girls were less physical, used softer language, and steered them towards playing with dolls, prams, and cuddly toys.

I was fascinated by this and it made me reflect on my relationship with my two boys and how I handled them, made contact with them, and played with them when they were younger. Before watching this programme, my view was that boys naturally and typically move towards a certain kind of behaviour and that their play is more externalised, with outward motion, bodily based, naturally taking risks and with more assertive behaviour, than is seen typically in girls. However, this programme, through research and experimentation, appeared to conclude that preferences were down to the external environment rather than biology.

It's all in the brain

This theory states that male and female brains are 'hardwired' differently. Neuroscience is in its infancy. It grabs headlines and makes bold extravagant claims. The controversial psychiatrist Louann Brizendine wrote a book called 'The Male Brain', in which she declares that the male brain has been 'marinated with testosterone' and is therefore hardwired, causing men to undertake risky behaviour, tell lies, and restrain their emotions. Her view could be summarised like this: men just can't help their behaviour, as that's how they are made.

Within her theory, there appears to be little space for brain development or growth and this, therefore, limits the expression of masculinity. This kind of thinking follows a long line of theories that seek to understand the differences between men and women in order to gain further assurance of gender differences. Yet when scans are made of baby's brains, it is impossible to spot any differences.

In 2015, a report entitled 'Male and female brains work the same way' based on a meta-analysis of seventy research papers, the result was inconclusive about any gender difference. According to the researchers,

> *'There is no difference in the size of the corpus callosum, white matter that allows the two sides of the brain to communicate, nor do men and women differ in the way their left and right hemispheres process language'.*[7]

However, much of this thinking is speculative, with certain theorists seeking to find the holy grail of gender difference and communicating this to the public as 'hard' knowledge. It might be more authentic to say, 'we don't know' and to lean on the wisdom of not-knowing and to accept that there are many different ways to express masculinity.

Perhaps, it would also be more helpful to communicate the 'soft' knowledge that we know: the brain has amazing plasticity, it absorbs an immense amount of information, and it has the ability to change as a result of environmental influences. As a result of the brain's plasticity, men are able to change and to modify their behaviour.

MEN ARE MADE THROUGH SOCIETAL MESSAGES

The societal instructions and nurturing of boys and girls is much easier to understand and essentially easier to change. I would like to highlight how society reinforces certain messages about boys and men and how these can harm boys/men and girls/women.

1. Male infants are shaped by gender socialisation and societal expectations

It's difficult for men not to be affected by family systems, religious systems, male role models, the media, and their peers. Men will constantly be receiving messages from the above sources that will be shaping their view of masculinity and how to act as a male. In a typical family, from day one when they are being held as a newly born baby, the language that is used towards male and female babies is different.

To a female it may be things like 'oh, isn't she beautiful, so lovely, so cute' and to a boy 'what a sturdy little chap', 'what a strong little boy', 'what a fighter'. As the boy grows up, he is immersed in this kind of language and the family messages which are communicated. From a very early age, boys are introduced to language and media which will give them strong hints as to what it means to be a boy. The gaming industry, films, magazines and toys have generated a powerful message for boys; these include what a boy should enjoy and what they should do to be a 'proper' boy.

As he grows up, the pressures to conform increase. The child may feel a desperate need to fit in. Gender has been commercialised and includes gender-specific colours such as pink and blue although in the Victorian era, girls were dressed in blue and boys in pink.

The gendering of products has become ridiculous. There are gender-specific male strong-edged crisps and chunky chocolate. Yorkie was marketed in 2002 with the slogan, 'It's not for girls'. There are even man-size tissues for men to cry big manly tears! A whole new range of male beauty products has emerged in recent years branded 'for men', as the other ones are clearly for women. Recently, I was given a gift — my first official man crème in a robust and well-designed little tin. Finally, I felt safe to moisturise while maintaining my masculinity!

2. Men are made by the 'Gender Break'

Being securely attached to a parent or significant adult is hugely important for any infant. It makes them feel safe, loved, affirmed, and confident in their identity. If an infant doesn't get this kind of affirming love, it could lead to them feeling unsafe, insecure and lacking grounding.

Later in life, they may display various behaviours to help them manage or cope with this 'lack of' in their life. For me personally, I had a lack of secure emotional attachment with my main carers and became heavily dependent on self-reliance and avoidant behaviour, which is still a default position I consciously have to challenge.

Vic Blake[8] coined the term 'Gender break', which describes another gender layer to the attachment theory. This concept seeks to describe the moment when boys become conscious that they have different genitalia to their main carer (typically the mother, female carer) and realise they are not the same.

This realisation can cause a kind of trauma, especially if the infant's father or other male figures are unavailable in terms of attention, time, affirmation, and affection. This event is very significant in the making of men, as it happens at a time when boys will be very conscious of the roles men play and what they can expect from men in their lives. The gender break creates a disruption and disturbance in the young boy's life and can contribute to complex developmental trauma.

3. Men are made through the trauma of emotional restriction

The trauma of emotional restriction is caused through developmental experiences that can have a hidden and increasingly obvious impact on the full development of boys. The typical boy will learn messages about masculinity and the expression of emotions very early on in his life. He learns that to be a man he will need to constantly prove himself worthy of being part of the male tribe by conforming to the male rules.

I will always recall an incident with my son when he was seven years old. He was hiding behind a hedge on our allotment, holding his knee with his face scrunched up in pain. He had already learnt the message on the playground, 'You will feel pain but you must not express it.'

You will feel pain but you must not express it

This is the core root of the trauma of emotional restriction and is a pre-cursor to the message, 'Big boys don't cry'. Like many boys, my son had realised the rules of physical and emotional pain and that to show or reveal vulnerable emotions on the playground is dangerous due to the risk of being humiliated and shamed. I have often heard this familiar story from boys about when they fall over, other boys are quick to point and laugh.

If the boy who is hurt dares to cry then he is hit with emotional shaming such as 'sissy', 'cry-baby', 'stop being a girl' and other similar phrases. This is the beginning of male emotional restriction that has been engineered through the 'male code' an unwritten list of rules that boys and men learn to live by described in a later chapter.

4. Men are made through the impact of individual experience and personality

The making of men will be influenced through their family of origin, family values and connection to their siblings. This personality or ego-state could be coded by sibling placement, early attachment issues, birthing issues and emotional or traumatic experiences. Different siblings of the same family will be unique in the way they perceive and experience the world, affecting how they express themselves.

Sibling placement may impact this in terms of how the male meets the world through introversion or extraversion. Family roles will also have an impact. In most family systems, children are given responsibility to be the 'perfect one', the 'problem one', the 'responsible one', the 'clown', the 'scapegoat, the 'favourite' one, the 'ill' one etc.

Trauma through implicit or explicit shaming within the family system, schooling or peers could also have shaped his expression of masculinity. It is important to acknowledge that boys develop parts of themselves at different stages. Growth and change are always possible.

What I am trying to demonstrate here is how ridiculous it is to say all men are the same, they are not. Being a man is indeed very complex and not just as simple as identifying genital difference or indeed size. The making of man is affected by each stage of his journey within the womb, his early attachments and experiences in the world.

CHAPTER 4:

A BRIEF HISTORY OF MANKIND

Only a few decades ago, many boys would work in the same industry as their fathers and perhaps join his business. His work would often be manual and he would learn a trade or skill and start his working life as an apprentice to a master craftsman. After years of watching, learning to handle tools and honing his skills, the boy would become a craftsman. He would have learnt to cherish and care for his tools and would know them intimately. His tools were essential for his survival.

After several more years of experience, he would earn the right to become a master craftsman. If today's boys want to become men, it is important they slow down, learn from the past, and take time to listen to the story of Mankind. This will be the beginning of change.

During the last fifty years, the world has drastically shifted. Many men feel left behind. The environment in which man finds himself has changed and it appears that on many levels, men have been finding it hard to adjust or evolve. It seems to be hurting them in untold ways.

Many commentators have suggested that masculinity is in crisis or that it is actually toxic, almost as if men are poisonous and there is something fundamentally wrong with them. Men and masculinity are on the national agenda more than ever before, but it is still rare for the state of man or of masculinity to be openly discussed.

In the UK, we have a minister for women but not a minister for men. We have a 'Woman's Hour' on Radio 4 but not a 'Men's Hour'. Some would say that men are so present and dominant in all major walks of life that it is not needed and yet, in my view, we desperately need to be talking about men in society, their changing roles, their impact, and the ways they are hurting.

THE 'M' WORD

Men have a high profile in society. They are in the media, on TV screens, on the news, and in power and positions of influence. We see them all the time, but we rarely talk about men and what it means to be a man in our society. When a spree killing occurs (usually perpetrated by a man) masculinity is never talked about. When a murder-suicide (a man kills family/strangers and then himself) happens in society, his masculinity is never mentioned.

When a boy stabs or shoots a teacher, the construction of his masculinity is never questioned. When the majority of prisoners are men and boys, the question of why this is the case is never asked. When a terrorist (usually men) drives a car into crowds and kills many innocent people, his gender is never mentioned. The media do not want or do not know, how to discuss masculinity and its shadow side. Clearly, in the above cases, I am highlighting a minority of men involved in these awful events. Not all men are like this, but the fact remains — it is mainly men perpetuating these crimes.

A man's gender is often invisible

In 2013, the Labour MP Diane Abbott gave a speech about masculinity and addressed some of the issues that men are facing. Subsequently, Abbot was criticised by a section of men involved in raising men's awareness, almost like how dare a woman talk about men's issues. Yet, in the speech she was able to name some difficulties that men are facing. Abbott said that the present male generation is 'caught between the 'stiff-upper-lip' approach of previous generations and today's cultural tornado of male cosmetics, white-collar industry, and modernised workplaces'.

If men are in crisis rather than in transition, then it may perhaps be because of entrenched views, inner hurts, and a lack of exploration in addressing how best to help men evolve. There are strong forces in society which refuse to allow men and boys to change. This may generate this perpetual crisis and a sense of unsettlement.

WHAT DOES IT MEAN TO BE A MAN?

Being a man used to be simple. The man's job was to be the protector and provider and the woman's role was to be the homemaker and nurturer. Unless you have been on a desert island, in prison, or lost in a forest for the past fifty years, you can't fail to see that the world isn't like that anymore.

Back then, you knew your place, you knew your role

Yet, I constantly hear men talking about being emasculated with women taking their jobs and roles in society and often expressing their insecurity through anger. These men are struggling to adapt and just want things to return to how they were. Back then, you knew where you were, things were black and white. Some men are struggling with the new era. Many men are struggling to adjust to the present reality. They feel a sense of nostalgia for the past, with its stricter gender roles.

THE GREAT MALE MIGRATION

The biggest invisible migration during the last sixty years has seen men's work situation changing, from manual work to mind work. This has brought a societal change: sixty years ago, the majority of men worked with their hands, they went to the factory, the pit and the land and they used their body, physical power and skill as their main way of earning a living. The rise in technology has meant that land work and factory work is increasingly being done by large vehicles and robots.

Pits have been closed and jobs have moved abroad. The migration began slowly but soon gathered pace with the invention of the computer. Men were moving indoors in vast numbers. They spent their days predominantly sitting down facing a computer screen and limited their body movements to exercising their fingers. Physical power was no longer essential, their body was no longer useful and their mind, thinking capacity and the ability to communicate were prized.

Men have traditionally always been good at thinking and using their rational and cognitive abilities, but many have failed to do the work on the inside of embracing their feelings or managing their mental fitness. Clearly, some men do still work in physical environments — professional sport relies on the body but the majority of men now work indoors in office environments.

Men's physical strength has increasingly become a redundant feature of their traditional role; they no longer need their body for physical survival. Within this sedentary culture in which obesity is an ever-increasing risk, men's physical exercise is also often indoors for example in a gym. Even their workout is now indoors.

Men's physical strength has increasingly become a redundant feature of their traditional role; they no longer need their body for physical survival

---

NEW MAN VERSUS NEW LADISM

Alongside societal changes, men have been seeking to change and work out what their role is, often in response to what is happening in culture. During the 1980s and early 1990s, things started to significantly change. Women were entering the workforce in far greater numbers. Increasingly, men and women were working together. Relational expectations were also changing. Some men became more domesticated and appeared 'softer' with the rise of the new man. Men adopting this stance started to share more of the housework, nurturing and assuming the responsibility for the children.

Masculinity confusion was very evident at this time with the rise of new ladism. This was a backlash to the 'new man' and took a 'boys will be boys' approach with enthusiasm about cars, womanising, and drinking. Ladism was supported by the 'lads' mag' culture. These magazines are essentially soft porn, alongside promoting general irresponsibility and a safe home for men who could not shift or accept the 'new man' masculinity. Video 'gaming' also became an important aspect for many lads.

Lads' magazines have clearly added to the confusing message about masculinity with mixed messages of useful health advice laced with familiar messages from the male code textbook. Ripped bodies, body mortification, meat eating, beer drinking, and increasing sexual conquests are often the staples of magazines aimed at men.

A BRIEF HISTORY OF MANKIND

1. **CAVE MAN** — He was a physical survivor and a hunter. He depended on fire, food, and sleep. (See Bear Grylls' TV programmes)
2. **ADVENTURER MAN** — The explorer. Men travelled to discover new lands and riches.
3. **CONQUEST MAN** — Colonial and conquering king. The strongest won dominion over 'weaker' races and power over others with the rise of patriarchy.
4. **WARRIOR MAN** — Fighting to be the top dog, the defender of 'right' and the age of world wars, weapons, and might.
5. **INDUSTRIAL MAN** — The technological man. Machine and man work in union to generate growth and wealth.
6. **POST-WAR MAN (1940s)** — The broken man and society. This period saw a questioning and re-establishing of gender male role positions in society.
7. **THE HIPPY/HOMOSEXUAL MAN (1960s)** — This period saw a questioning of power, war, and authoritarian discourses. Men were involved in generating free love, peace, and questioning sexual constraints. In this period, men began to accept and show love to each other. In 1967, homosexual acts in private between two men both aged twenty-one and over were decriminalised.

8. **POST-INDUSTRIAL MAN (LATE 1980s)** — The loss of traditional outdoor male jobs, loss of traditional working patterns, loss of jobs for life. Work security was starting to erode with the age of redundant men.

9. **THE NEW MAN** — In the 1990s, the new, softer, more domesticated man and father starts to emerge, alongside the backlash of 'ladism' and the lad's magazines.

10. **METROSEXUAL MAN** — A term coined by Mark Simpson[9] to describe the cosmetic commercial potential of the urban, sophisticated, self-care man. David Beckham is a good example of the metrosexual. Alongside this, the Retro-sexual man battled for the old ways of traditional man to be observed.

11. **LUMBERSEXUAL MAN (2005ish)** — The hipster urban male with large facial hair and checked shirts. The latest emerging male fashion seeking to re-wild men.

12. **GENTROSEXUAL MAN (2013)** — As proposed by FHM men's magazine. A decent guy with manners, a family man, successful and 'is more likely to stop a fight than start one'. (Top example = Ryan Gosling)

13. **SPORNOSEXUAL MAN (2015)** — Another term coined by Mark Simpson[10] to describe the man who has been inspired by the sporting and porn industries. Men like this typically enjoy revealing toned, ripped and sculpted physics with little body hair. (Top example = footballer Cristiano Ronaldo)

THE METRO-SEXUAL VERSUS THE RETRO-SEXUAL

In 1994, Mark Simpson coined the term 'Metro Sexual' to describe the latest commercial endeavour to open up a new market of male grooming and care products. The modern, urban man's fascination with his appearance and narcissistic lifestyle had opened up new ways of expressing masculinity. Male models in magazines often appeared androgynous. This created uncomfortable questions about masculinity.

In 2008, Dave Beasley wrote a humorous book entitled, 'The Retrosexual Manual — How to be a Real Man'. This was written in direct response to the metro-sexualisation of men and wanting men to return to the 1970s when a man could 'really be a man'. This is a book wishing that things could return to how they were and fearing that men have been emasculated. Beasley wrote:

> *They've taken away our language, our clothes, our pubs, our cars, even our confidence — our very essence of manliness.'* [11]

The retrosexual is defined by the male code. It is a plea, coming from an insecure masculinity with the warrior cry 'they have emasculated us', which will be explored later in this book.

THE GENTROSEXUAL AND LUMBERSEXUAL

Around 2013, the 'Lumbersexual man' emerged as the latest fashion inspired expression of modern masculinity. Facial hair in the style of a big, manicured bushy beard was back in and no self-respecting hipster would be without one. This well-dressed man would sport boots and possibly a flannel-style shirt. This fashion display sought to transmit the rugged wild outdoors man alongside the sophistication of the modern, urban man.

Also in 2013, the magazine entitled FHM suggested that the Gentrosexual[12] is the new modern man, describing him in terms of attitudes rather than looks. FHM surveyed their readers to discover modern male attitudes. This is what they found:

- 69% of FHM readers said that male roles in society had changed in the last 15 years
- 96% of readers would not object if a premier league footballer came out as gay
- 98% believe it is important to have good manners
- 7% of guys believe that cooking is solely a women's responsibility
- 93% of men think getting into fights for trivial reasons is dumb

Clearly, these results represent a small demographic and percentage of men and yet in many ways, this survey about modern masculinity should be welcomed. It reveals some positive results and insights. On the downside, however, there appears little evidence in this survey that men have expanded their expression of emotion and they continue to find it difficult to challenge the 'rules' that constrain men's emotional evolvement.

WHAT ABOUT HER STORY?

Perhaps it is impossible for men to evolve psychologically if they don't spend time contemplating the story of women in history. Can we understand men without reflecting on the historical story of women and the prescribed roles of men and women? HIS story has roles for men and women. HIS story has been told and written into the history books by powerful, wealthy and successful men.

HER story has rarely been heard or recorded in the history books. Her-story has often been hidden and silenced and when she has been written about she has often been accused of HEResy. Women have been derided, tortured, raped, murdered, accused of being witches, excluded from political systems and careers, and often paid less than men for doing an equivalent job.

Yet, during the last century with hard-won freedoms and the battle for equality, it is women who have evolved, changed and adapted, and ultimately become future-focused. During this time, men appear to have conceded and adapted to the present situation but have struggled to embrace true change. Many men feel that they have been doing all the 'giving' and the letting go. As a result, some feel resentful of the situation as it currently stands.

Most men live in male-centric societies and often remain blind to male privilege and bias. Many men concede and adapt to gender equality reluctantly and externally, resulting in a lack of desire for change, limiting integral internal movement

---

Some men are left wondering what the pay-off is for them, what do they get in return. Some men view gender equality as a loss or as an act of empowerment. The problem with empowerment is that the powerful do the empowering. In essence, they still hold the power. Personally, it has been hard for me to become aware of my male-centric position, views, and behaviour and I often feel I have only just begun the journey.

I have learnt a lot about what it means to live as a woman in this world through my wife, female colleagues, friends, and clients. There are so many things I am unable to notice as a man that many women just adapt to. It is a bit like living as a homosexual in a heteronormative society.

The world is seen from a heterosexual point of view with blissful unawareness of what homosexuals have to endure. When women have the courage to challenge the status quo, question misogyny, seek equality, and assert themselves, some men will respond with aggressiveness and passive-aggressive behaviour.

Men may feel their freedom and way of being is encroached upon and eroded when women want to infiltrate or question the old boys' network and the status quo. My wife has expressed how exhausting it is to move from a place of passive acceptance to asserting her rights as a woman and essentially as a human. For men to grow and develop, it is essential that we listen to women's stories and learn to understand and empathise with their worldview and experience.

Societal male privilege and a lack of equality is actually harming men

It is still a man's world. Men enjoy the most privilege, hold on to the majority of senior positions and have greater power. Even in my own profession of psychotherapy, the hierarchy is very evident. It is mainly men who developed the popular psychotherapeutic modalities and yet my profession is mostly populated by women.

When I attend therapeutic courses, it is quite normal that I am the only male on the course, however, the majority of books on Psychotherapy are written by men and many of the training courses are taught by men.

The lack of equality in the workplace and men's need for achievement is essentially harming men's physical and emotional health. Their inner drive to succeed at all costs is causing men to die younger. The leading causes of death for men are suicide, heart disease, cancer, and strokes. Men often hold onto so much pressure and stress that their body cannot absorb any more.

'Suicide kills more people then stomach cancer, breast cancer, colon cancer and Alzheimer's.'

— WORLD HEALTH ORGANISATION[13]

Suicide is the leading cause of death of men under 35

True gender equality is healthy for all sexes. Men will become healthier and happier when they live in a society that can fully embrace these fundamental changes.

FUTURISTIC MAN

In this brief journey through the story of masculinity, it is evident the present situation is harming men and hindering growth. Ancient roles and archetypes for the modern man are largely redundant. In terms of change, men have often been reactive rather than proactive. Movement has remained cosmetic rather than internal.

Men have often been clinging onto old internal ways of being whilst being busy upgrading appearance and new technology. This has often left men removed from their internal senses, hindering intimacy and growth. Societal change during the previous sixty years has been an uncomfortable and anxious ridden journey for many boys and men. Men have often lacked role models who have confidently shown them what modern masculinity is and what lies at the core of a secure manhood.

**Boys and men often feel lost.
They are left to struggle in isolation and fear**

If we are going to learn from the history of masculinity, we need to listen to the past, stop being reactive and start being more proactive. Men need to change, but they must see the value in changing. My view is that men must do the hard, painful work of embracing their emotions and feeling their feelings. If they don't, they will be perpetually sucked back into a place of stunted development. They will be fearful that they are being emasculated.

What I intend to show in this book is that men need to make the transition into 'Emosexual', where they will be able to embrace the full spectrum of emotions. In the future, men will need to move from merely surviving to thriving and this will be an internal job. Could the story of mankind be challenged and changed through men becoming kinder to themselves?

CHAPTER 5:
THE RISE OF THE KIDULT

'When a population becomes distracted by trivia, when cultural life is redefined as a perpetual round of entertainments, when serious public conversation becomes a form of baby-talk, when, in short, a people become an audience and their public business a vaudeville act, then a nation finds itself at risk; culture-death is a clear possibility.'

— NEIL POSTMAN[14]

Many men love their tools. They love shiny new gadgets, technology, and video games. They like to own the latest sports gear. They will spend hours researching the top equipment and enjoy looking good in the right gear.

Occasionally, I find myself feeling a little superior and inwardly proud when I go on a public golf course (it happens about once every five years). I turn up with a few old clubs and appear to do better than the bloke with the radio-controlled golf bag, latest fashion wear, and top of the range set of clubs.

We do appear to live in an age where men are keen to have the latest and best tools for the job but may not spend so much time learning how to use them, respect them and look after them. Perhaps for men to grow up, they need to spend more time learning their trade and practising using their emotional tools. What state are their emotional tools in?

When did they last clean them and sharpen them? This chapter describes how men have been prevented from growing up.

THE POWER OF THE BOY

I was a late developer. I was late having sex, late getting married, late having children, late having any financial security, and late in growing up emotionally. For the first thirty-five years of my life, I felt like a boy. I was a boy trapped inside a man's body.

The boy parts of me still needed something, they still needed to be parented, to be affirmed and loved and without these needs being met, the 'boy' dominated my life. I carried a huge amount of shame. I disliked myself. I feared others and how they might humiliate, embarrass, and expose me.

I was a fragile human being, constantly comparing myself with others and regularly beating myself up emotionally. I was a Kidult!

It wasn't until I could admit to myself and literally verbalise out loud how utterly 'fucked up' I was that I reached a kind of threshold. After all the years of hiding behind my ego and the pretence of being mature and together, I had come to the realisation I was lying to myself and the world around me.

It wasn't until I hit painful conflict and suffered burnout that I began the journey of waking up. I literally went on retreat for three years at the 'Northumbria community', where I was able to face myself, indulge in frightening soul searching, and finally be ruthlessly honest with myself.

I was able to face my incongruent self and begin embracing the truth of how I really felt.

Having been brought up in a strict religious household and culture, to actually shout out loud that I was 'fucked up' felt like another milestone and a transitional moment. This was no doubt one of the most difficult stages of my life, in which I felt lost, alone, weak, and not knowing where this journey would lead. It was, however, the period which started to help me to grow up and wake up to how the interior life was such an unknown territory to me.

ADULTLESCENCE

Gary Cross, an American academic and researcher, has written an in-depth analysis of the delayed development of men. He suggests men have been locked into a 'Peter Pan syndrome' in his excellent book entitled 'Men to Boys — The Making of Modern Immaturity'. He coins the term 'adultlesence' as a way of describing many men who have become kidults, boy-men or adult-boys and become stuck in an extended adolescence.

Cross explores how he feels that the infantilisation of men is evident and the infiltration of the porn industry into many areas of society, essentially promoting women as play things and men as sex machines (the playboy). This male infantilisation can also be observed in gadget man, pal dads and the rise of the metro-sexual.

Cross suggests that the metro-sexual and the look that accompanies it may be about preserving the cherished childhood, removing body hair and seeking to preserve the pre-pubescent look. Cross writes: *'It is no surprise that men stuck in the emotional life of a teenager would try to make themselves more physically boy-like'.*[15]

The adult boy is stuck in a state in which he needs more, needs it to be bigger, is a thrill-seeker, likes it fast, is always 'on', and struggles to develop regulation or responsibility. Cross continues, '*The boy-man stands on the treadmill of endless novelty and passively looks for 'hits' of pleasure while the adult man cultivates, savours and gives back*'.[16]

This 'Peter Pan Syndrome' which many men are locked into exhibits itself through being fun, charming, and successful. But ultimately, there is an emotional immaturity in which they are unable to handle love or responsibility. The world glorifies the boys. Sports cars, action movies, games that indulge male fantasy, pornography, advertising, football culture — all of it plays to the male preoccupation with winning, playing, and youthful images of virility.

JUST PLAY

Familiar refrains that men may often hear from women include phrases such as: 'When are you going to grow up?' 'He's just a kid at heart.' 'It's like I live with three boys.'

There is no doubt that boys and men love playing, as it is a key way they have learnt to make contact. Playing sports, gaming, or collecting has become an important way of men connecting with others or with themselves. However, one question that is important to address is this: does this 'need to play' hinder them from growing up?

As boys grow into adults their tastes for toys just becomes more expensive with the financial ability to increase their haul

---

This behaviour is regarded as acceptable and it appears men are quite comfortable with the 'boys and their toys' term to describe their collective obsession with gadgets, cars, and big watches.

Not only have men continued to play games but it has also been turned into a global business. What used to be just for enjoyment has been legitimised into a way of making a large amount of money. The gaming industry is now a multi-billion-dollar entity, mainly directed towards and appealing to men and boys. The games include sport, violent adventure, action hero, shooting, conquest games, and speed where the values of winning, power and competition are central. Online games now boast players belonging to clans. The top groups are making BIG money.

The nerds have taken over the world

Gaming has become incredibly lucrative for the men who were once bullied for being nerds. But gaming has grown and now invades modern life. Boys and men spend hours and hours in front of screens playing games. The amount of screen time has risen from two hours a day (in 2013) to as much as eight hours a day now. Screen-based media is also causing much concern, as it leads to isolation and a sedentary lifestyle, which may also be contributing to the obesity epidemic and possible future posture issues.

There is also concern that boys and men are showing signs of addictive behaviour and questions have been raised about how the content of the games is affecting their social skills, management of conflict, and emotional regulation. I have heard many teenage boys' stories of how they can be gaming for up to sixty hours a week, including sessions going through the night. One boy I worked with told me how, at the weekend, he plays on the Xbox with his brother and father. They do this by each sitting in their own bedroom with their own console and screen and playing each other online all weekend, only stopping occasionally to eat.

Sport, supported by the media boom, has also been turned into a huge business, where a boyhood pursuit and dream can now reap huge amounts of wealth.

The significance of sport and the power of sport are quite extraordinary to observe

---

Nations are devoted to their national sport. Results make headline news often affecting a nation's psyche. The 2018 football World Cup produced euphoria in the UK and elsewhere. Sport is no longer just a game, it's not just little boys' stuff. Playing with balls, kicking, hitting, throwing or catching is now a very serious and important commodity. As a business, it is dominated by men at all levels. The men's game is taken much more seriously and is typically much more important than women's sport. However, recently women's sport has been gaining a larger profile in sports such as football, cricket, and rugby.

Stibbe (2004) in his critique of Men's Health magazine believes that sport promotes hegemonic masculinity and a masculine agenda of power. Stibbe quotes from the magazine about the benefit of watching hockey brawls:

> *'If we didn't have them we'd resort to more destructive behaviour, like sharing our feelings'.*[17]

This bizarre statement shows how hard it is for men to share and verbalise their feelings. Do men actually perceive feelings as destructive? Is this one of the reasons why men fear feelings?

MEN ONLY ZONES

Most boys and men enjoy spending time together. Boys have learnt that they need a reason to hang out together. Being together is not enough and they need to be doing something together. Before screens, boys would create dens together, build go-karts and have adventures, experiment and devise imaginary play. Much of boys' play today takes place within painted lines on the ground and governed by adult supervisors.

As boys grow into men, they can still find themselves wanting to inhabit men only zones. Sports clubs offer this and some golf clubs in the UK still operate male-only membership. Religion still offers male-only zones. Men still create and hold onto male-only societies such as clubs like the Masons, working men's clubs and private 'smoking' men's clubs. It is fair to say, some of these organisations have more recently created women's sections and allowed women to join the club. However, men continue to be the main gender indulging in hobbies such as stamp, toy, and games collection, steam train enthusiasm and war enactments.

Cross suggests, *'Hobbies offered men a chance to share a boy-man world of escape from the expectations of maturity, even in neglecting child rearing... a perfect expression of nostalgia and an escape from adult responsibility.'*[18]

Not only do men tend to have clubs and hobbies that particularly attract just men, they also like to create men-only zones that they can inhabit alone or with the lads. As mentioned earlier many men like to think of certain spaces as 'their' space such as the shed, garage, and basement, cellar, or loft. It is their space where they can be messier, cooler, and wilder.

Why are these men-only zones so important for men? What needs do they meet? Cross wonders if there is perhaps a strong psychological element to this common occurrence. He suggests boys learn that their early identification with their mother is shameful. Boys hear many shaming messages such as 'acting like a girl' and 'mummy's boy'.

These messages can be amplified if boys have a cold, distant, or driven father. It is almost as if Men Only Zones are useful to bolster masculinity, to help boys and men understand the rules and learn to play competitively. This stage is often plain to see in the push-pull relationship played out between teenage boys and their mothers. The boy is caught between showing love and protection for his mother and on the playground responding to 'your mum' insults.

Then at home he is involved in a struggle to become more independent, to be his own person and part of this process necessitates pushing Mum away. In modern society, this can often include some form of verbal abuse. Cross suggests that some men continue to play this game on the world stage and will seek to steer away from 'sissy' politics to avoid their masculinity being called into question.

'Masculinity is a hard won, yet precious and brittle psychological achievement that must be constantly proven and defended.'[19]

RITES OF PASSAGE

A rite of passage is an ancient tradition practised in many tribes all over the world. The essential belief of this ancient rite is that boys need to go through a physical process to help them make the transition into becoming a man. There can be several rites of passage or transitional phases throughout a person's life. In modern society, however, we pay little attention to this despite its significance.

Puberty is the core rite of passage. It includes a paradigm shift in body, brain, and emotional development. The young person will receive a massive injection of chemicals that will surge through their system essentially rewiring their brains. As you can imagine, this will and should have a significant impact on the young person, as the biological pattern prepares the individual to enter the next stage of their life.

In many modern societies, we ultimately leave girls and boys to go through this phase in isolation. Girls are left to deal with menstruation and boys with their wet dreams alone. They are being left to deal with potentially unspoken shame on their own. If these things are not addressed and they usually aren't, the adolescent does not know how to address the physical changes they are encountering or the challenging concurring emotions.

Traditional rites of passage include three phases. The first stage is separation. In this stage, the individual is typically removed from the tribe or the group to signify that the person is about to enter a new phase in their life. In some tribal situations, there could be a mock 'kidnapping' of the boy from the mother to symbolically demonstrate the cutting away or removal of the earlier stage of life and the movement to the next stage.

The middle stage is called the liminal or in-between phase. Typically, in traditional rites of passage this stage would include certain tests, education of new tribal responsibilities, and preparation for the next stage of life. This test may include learning to survive in the wild for several days alone with limited supplies. The test is a 'toughening' up experience to enhance the boy's ability to fend for himself and be a good warrior.

The third and final stage is reincorporation into the tribe. The individual is celebrated and welcomed back having completed the 'rite' and taken on their new identity. At this stage, with a sense of becoming a new person, the man may be given a new name and a different role. Ties will have been strengthened and respect is given.

The person enduring the 'rite' has now been given full membership of their group; they are fully incorporated into the mature levels of that society. Of course, the girls of the tribe will also have to experience a rite of passage which will often include enduring pain.

Richard Rohr has studied male rites of passage, examining the process in many traditional tribal societies. He believes five messages are taught during the liminal stage and these help to prepare the boy for the next stage of life. The five messages are counter-cultural and as follows:

1. **Life is hard.** If you can accept this early on, it will help to prevent meaningless pain and waste of time in the future.
2. **You are going to die.** Different parts/stages of your life will need to die or to be left behind before you can move onto the next stage.
3. **You are not that important.** Embracing humility and smallness and questioning the power of the ego-state is a crucial stage in practising empathy and interconnectedness.
4. **You are not in control.** This is a vital message to learn in order to adjust to acceptance of other people and in learning emotional awareness. The paradox of control is that less is more.
5. **Your life is not about you.** This is a message about interconnectedness of all things, society, family, the other and the greater good. We are a part of something bigger.[20]

You may feel these messages are negative. Within an individualistic mindset, this is how they can be perceived. But without the provision of a rite of passage for communicating these messages, boys and men can be lost in a crisis and are desperately left to look for a tribal or gender sense of belonging in other places, including gang culture, drugs, fraternity groups and sports membership.

Some modern organisations that offer rites of passage for boys and men believe that 'boys are born and men are made' and therefore it is essential that boys are modelled an 'authentic masculine' way of being. The old African proverb, 'it takes a whole village to raise a child.' makes a lot of sense.

In my own study and formulation of ancient and modern rites of passage, I have concluded that the loss of marking different stages of life can hinder successful transitions. Ancient tribal rites were important as ways of passing on cultural traditions. They appeared to be an important part of the survival of the people group. Modern rites may include raising issues regarding global survival and incorporate more physiological and psychological elements such as identity formation, social responsibility, environmental interconnectedness, community and emotional fitness.

Perhaps a lack of modern rites of passage is prolonging the life of the boy and preventing him from growing up, acting his age is not the problem, growing up is

---

Does a lack of formal rites of passage for boys and girls within modern culture have an adverse effect on them? If rites are not created and modelled within modern cultures by the 'elders' then will young people seek to do it for themselves? They may use dysfunctional methods such as self-harming. These and other questions are important ones to ask when there seems to be many pseudo ways of doing this in present society.

PSEUDO RITES OF PASSAGE

Many of the pseudo-rites have a commonality with the past in that they are based on brutality and shaming within a hierarchical system. These practices exist in a number of ways including gang initiation, rugby club initiation, belonging to university fraternities, and industrial-scale bullying such as hazing. Hazing is an American term for brutal initiation tests in military establishments. Boarding schools have also been places that have operated brutal pseudo rites of passage within their hierarchical structures of their student population.

Jeremy Clarkson, who became famous for being on the 'Top Gear' BBC programme. Clarkson wrote an article in the Independent newspaper, focusing on his experience of boarding school. He wrote how, when he was at boarding school, he was mercilessly bullied:

> *"As the years dragged by I suffered many terrible things, I was thrown on an hourly basis into the icy plunge pool, dragged from my bed in the middle of the night and beaten. I was made to lick the lavatories clean and all the usual humiliations that public school used back then to turn a small boy into a gibbering, sobbing suicidal wreck".*[21]

This account is deeply disturbing. It explains some of Clarkson's trauma, public antics, heartlessness, outspoken comments and behaviour towards some of the people who worked with him. The mentality of 'Top Gear' was kidult. They were mates, but they constantly belittled each other and put each other down. Perhaps he has not been able to deal with that childhood pain and is transmitting it onto others.

The story of Clarkson's traumatic time at school reveals how many boys implicitly feel and show how they develop their emotional armour in order to survive an often physical and psychologically traumatic period of their lives.

Apprenticeships traditionally were the basis for how young family members learnt their fathers' trade and more recently businesses provided these to train young boys in manual skills. When I was sixteen, I began an apprenticeship in carpentry and joinery and entered the world of working men. In many ways, this was a rite of passage and included doing the 'dirty jobs', being tricked and sometimes humiliated and shamed. I think in many ways I got off lightly, but I can remember often returning home feeling scared and in tears.

In recent years, many more young people have been entering the world of university. There is an ongoing debate which asks whether university prolongs adolescence. Young people leave home and move into accommodation with a mono-aged community, to study their chosen subject and have a huge amount of freedom. For some people, this can mean they enter a world of over-consumption in drink, drugs and sex, which is readily available within town centres in every city in the country.

Many of these young people are clearly longing to get away from the restrictions of home, but have not yet developed self-regulation. It is almost as if their lives have become so sanitised, boring and life zapping that they long for wildness. This wildness is conjured up through 'party culture' with the aid of substances and can often end in recklessness, remorse and regret. In the UK, many university counselling services are struggling to manage the influx of students who are presenting with a variety of emotional issues and behaviours including anxiety, depression, isolation, and self-harm.

If these transitional phases in life aren't recognised, then perhaps this could be one of the causes of young people struggling to move through the different stages of life. The lack of the 'cutting away' stage has left young people feeling more susceptible to feeling alone, isolated and cut off from a community. In a more individualistic society with young people spending more time inside, isolated and perusing social media, they may have lost touch with the bigger picture.

IN AND OUT OF THE ARMY

When military environments fail to recognise the stages of transition and the importance of these then young men are left unprepared for the impact of these changes. They use the old tools in 'uniforming' civilians into another tribe, but provide little support when veterans, some of whom have spent years in an institution, re-enter the civilian tribe and start a different stage of their life.

Many of these ex-soldiers leave the army with mental health problems and alcohol problems, causing addiction and homelessness or they wind up in another institution, usually prison.

COMING OUT OF THE MILITARY

Charlie was in his early thirties and had been in the army for all his adult life. He was angry. He was advised to come to see me because his aggression was getting him into trouble and affecting his relationship.

At home, he would shout and smash things in violent rages. On the streets, if someone looked at him 'funny', he would have to hit the other guy. Now he was getting into trouble with the police. He showed no remorse, was defensive and did not want to address his problems. He was struggling to adjust to civilian life. He could only identify with his brothers in arms. He would often say, 'civilians had no idea what I have been through'. He prided himself that deep down, he was a better person than mere civilians. Sometimes, he needed to prove it.

My sense was that he was struggling with the transition from army to civilian life and adjusting to a life where his awareness of 'threat' didn't need to be permanently switched 'on'. Charlie had been conditioned to be vigilant against any physical threat and alert to any perceived emotional threat against his fragile state. In therapy, he was resistant, combative and defensive. He was not ready. After a couple of sessions, he pulled out.

After about six months, Charlie contacted me again. He had been in a lot more trouble due to his violent behaviour and there was a real chance that he would go to prison. He was different; he had begun to mellow and appeared to be taking responsibility for his behaviour and language. He was ready to do some emotional work and start the process of facing some of his emotional wounds. Therapy became a transitional place for him, almost like a rite of passage.

Together, we explored how his experiences as a boy and his conditioning within the army was driving him to behave in an aggressive way. He became aware of what was happening internally. I provided a safe space for Charlie to talk about his vulnerability and experience the right emotions at the right time. He was able to change and was in a very different place when he left therapy.

AN EMOTIONAL RITE OF PASSAGE

In ancient times, the rite of passage was something societies felt was helpful for guiding boys and girls through a stage of life where they had to leave childhood behind and take on responsibility for the tribe and assume a role in their society. Industrialisation disrupted family groups, community traditions, and natural family apprenticeships into the father's trade. Institutional religions, sport, gangs, and militarisation have all filled this transitional void.

Today, many of the old institutions and rites of passage have disappeared. Many young people feel lost. Alongside this, the breakdown of extended family networks and nuclear family disintegration has left more and more young people isolated and struggling to find their way. This has generated an increase in the adult boys stuck in comfort zones and unable to grow up.

To finally grow up and move away from the domination of the boy will demand that men begin to take themselves through an emotional rite of passage. When men chose to enter this kind of rite, they will be on the road to adjusting, changing and evolving. This shift takes courage, discipline, and training. If men refuse this journey, then they risk being the perpetual boy.

If the boy does not grow up, he will have a midlife crisis

Another crucial passage that confuses many men and can cause a 'crisis' is the 'middle' passage of life, classically between the ages of thirty-five and fifty-five. I am transitioning through the middle passage of life and moving into the second half of life and I am noticing how this affects me physically and psychologically.

If we accept and work with the changes this can be a fruitful and beautiful experience, but if men resist or avoid it, it can then turn into a midlife crisis. When the middle-aged man refuses to accept this physical and emotional transition, they are at risk of lurching back into the past, in a desperate hope of hanging onto their youth and the 'boy'.

The future looks scary and letting go is too painful to embrace

Welcoming the second stage of life and embracing the changes and beauty that age brings, can be a real opportunity for growth. One part of this stage for my wife and me was moving through the transition from being able to conceive children to moving beyond this and marking this stage of our lives by acknowledging this with a written ritual. Part of embracing this transition was my willingness to end the ability to reproduce by choosing to have a vasectomy.

While this was an insignificant physical procedure to undergo, it was a much bigger psychological procedure to consider. I was electing to give up the possibility of having more children. I have included some of the words spoken that I wrote for our intimate ceremony. We used these words to articulate the change in our lives. We spoke the words together.

It has been a privilege to co-create life. To be the instrument and incubator of our beautiful boys who have brought us so much joy and frustration. They continue to bless us with their presence and teach us so much about life, the unknown, and ourselves.

Alone and together, we have made the decision not to seek to produce further children and we consciously and willingly let go of this stage of our lives.

Together we let go of the potential to create a new life, together we let go of the potential of giving birth to a daughter and the time for biological birthing has ended.

These words helped us to articulate our sadness and a willingness to let go of hopes and dreams. We were acknowledging this season of our life was over.

If a man has not done some emotional growing before the age of thirty-five, there is a strong likelihood he will experience a mid-life crisis rather than taking the mid-life passage that will lead to the second half of life.

THE KIDULT TEST!

Men, take the kidult test. Women, do it for the men in your life. How many of the following statements are true for him?

1. Likes to be with the lads: spends more than two nights and half a day with them.
2. Ideal job working in a male environment where he can have a laugh: Typical male-centric employment including sports, sex industry, construction, banking, etc.
3. Plays sports or follows a team constantly, spending money and time following his team passionately at the cost of other relationships.
4. Has an all-consuming hobby which could include fishing, computers, cars, collecting various objects.
5. Plays screen (video) games for over 8 hours a week.
6. Owns many electronic gadgets including the latest toys, sports gizmos, and other 'really useful' must-have stuff.
7. Enjoys talking about and spending lots of time and money on cars.
8. Takes little responsibility for domestic chores — under 45% of tasks.
9. Is unable to cook.
10. Is unable to do his washing or ironing.
11. Very rarely apologises for mistakes.

12. Is driven by status and achievement.
13. Understands wealth as a sign of status.
14. Excessive bodybuilder.
15. Uses sexist language.
16. Uses homophobic language.
17. Communicates by banter, putting others down, making fun of them, mocking, belittling, verbal bullying (as against a friendly banter).
18. Treats women like objects (whistles, ogling, thinking about what he would like to do to her).
19. Sexually addictive — uses pornography, ogling at pictures of women in papers, lads' magazines etc.
20. Uses phrases like 'the missus', 'her', 'women are like...', 'she is doing my head in'.
21. Physically and verbally aggressive.
22. Regularly has to watch several TV sports for over 10 hours a week.
23. Spends little time with his children — apart from playing screen games or other passive activities.
24. If he is not living with his child, he will contribute little time and financially to the child's upbringing. (I am aware this is a complex issue for many men not living with their children — I am describing men with little intent).

25. Displays little empathy for others: laughs at, humiliates and ridicules others rather than thinking of the other's feelings/ situation.

26. Lack of communication skills — struggles to listen to others.

27. Emotionally illiterate — doesn't share his feelings.

28. Workaholic — spends more than 60 hours at work a week including travelling.

29. Addicted to a substance including alcohol, nicotine, caffeine, cannabis, or other drugs.

30. Defensive — attacks anyone who may question his lifestyle by being defensive, through denial or projecting the issue onto others.

31. Adrenaline junkie-addiction to speed, high-risk sports.

IS HE ACTING HIS AGE?

If he scored 20-31 — he is stuck in his boy and needs to seriously grow up.

If he scored 11-19 — he is a teenager boy and it's time to stop the wet dreams.

If he scored 5-10 — he is still holding onto teenager status and needs to have courage to take responsibility for himself. Time to stop the tantrums.

If he scored 1-4 — sounds like he has the making of being a responsible man.

CHAPTER 6:

THE MAN RULES — THE TERMS AND CONDITIONS OF BEING MALE

The man rules are what cultural observers have identified as the common stereotypical traits passed down from one generation of men to the next. These unspoken and unwritten rules will be known by the majority of men. They learnt them from their fathers, mothers, society, media, and peers. The man rules (also known as the male code) are like the small print within the terms and conditions of being male. Once learnt, men are expected to place a tick in the small box and forever stick to the code. If he fails to abide by the agreed terms and conditions then he can expect the full weight of humiliation to come upon him.

Women have, of course, also been given a code of conduct through the same channels. These culturally sanctioned codes of conduct become the norm and inform societal views of gender differentiation and are used as a typical baseline for how masculinity and femininity is described and understood.

Ron Levant in his book, 'Masculinity Reconstructed'[22] wrote down the male code after many years of research in working with men. The rules appear to be natural and instinctual and yet they have been framed as a way for men to keep their identity and mystique intact. It essentially creates a hierarchy of masculinity. If you are an 'alpha' male, then you will be better at abiding to the rules to a higher standard which then propels you up the pecking order.

To keep men in check and abiding by the rules, shame is the concealed weapon of choice sheathed in the scabbard of the 'The Real Man' discourse

Maintaining the rules is tiring, ultimately an incongruous activity and essentially makes masculinity a very slippery concept in which men have to constantly remain vigilant and always be ready to prove themselves. Levant proposed seven norms that will be briefly outlined below. In part three of the book, we will consider these in much more depth.

RULE #1 — AVOID ALL THINGS FEMININE

'What does it mean to be a man?' is a question I will often ask men who attend the groups I facilitate. This question is also one often posted on internet debates and highlights the fragility that many men feel about masculinity. Many men will answer this question with typical responses like 'being strong', 'being tough' or 'staying in control'.

Men I have worked with have answered this question by responding with 'not being a woman'. They define masculinity by separating themselves from any similarities to women, making sure that their gender cannot be confused with anything feminine.

Stereotypically women are seen as soft and moist, linked to genitalia but men should be hard and rigid, showing no signs of penetration or weakness. This becomes clear when we listen to male banter or abuse of other men. Men will call other men a 'wuss', 'a girl', 'soft' and say 'stop acting/crying like a girl'. To be a man, he must show no signs that the way he behaves can have any connection with stereotypical female behaviour.

In the past, women were perceived as weak due to several behaviours including their ability to express their emotions. To be associated with a female is shaming. If he wants to be a man and if he has to be strong and not show any sign of weakness, then he must restrict emotional expression, which isn't that difficult because he learnt these rules as a boy. To belong to 'A' grade masculinity, he must act rationally and always be in control.

This rule can affect men's relationships with their mother, partner, and daughter. His behaviour may change whilst in their presence. There are so many complexities associated within these relationships including the need to reinforce the male rule and seek to 'be the man'. Men will often feel the need to live up to this rule living in fear that a female could man-shame them. The boy will have learnt how to stay relatively safe in male specific groups and activities.

RULE #2 — RESTRICT ONE'S EMOTIONAL LIFE

Emotional restriction is one of the key lessons boys have learnt early on in their lives. It takes time to unlearn such a powerful protective coping strategy. The first rule also reinforced this through shame-based behaviour of being associated with girls or indeed babies.

Because of this second rule, men's spectrum of emotional expression has been severely curtailed, leaving them with limited tools to express what is going on inside them. Often men are just left with anger as a way of expressing themselves. This impacts on relationships in many ways. This rule has taught men to live inside their heads and essentially makes them emotionally mute.

They are left to suffer from alexithymia (a lack of emotional language to express their feelings) and this eventually inhibits their growth and can ultimately harm men, physically and emotionally. They have learnt not to express pain and not to ask for help and this rule is killing men.

Taught to isolate themselves, they are in danger of keeping shameful and difficult feelings inside themselves. This can contribute to mental health issues, self-harm, and even suicide.

RULE #3 — EMPHASIZE ACHIEVING STATUS ABOVE ALL ELSE

One of the lessons boys learnt from men is: men are big and the bigger you are, the more respect you will command. Often boys will lack affirmation and approval from their father, yet they deeply long for it.

In my therapeutic practice, I have lost count of the boys and men who have indicated they have never received a 'well done' or a positive comment from their father. A classic example of this would be when a boy returns with his exam results and they are all 'A's apart from one grade. The father chooses to focus on the 'B' and does not offer any positive feedback. Mothers can also demand that their son is perfect. At this age, boys learn they need to constantly prove themselves, work hard, become successful, and get to the top of the pile.

Boys learn the message, 'winning is all there is' and being the biggest and best is the way to find their place in the slippery world of masculinity. This approach may generate addiction to work and being successful in business with little thought about family and relationships. A ruthless approach to make sure his status is secure. The pressure of this approach to life and work is very stressful and sometimes overwhelming. Often, this attitude and way of working is driven by a deep psychologically unmet need.

Status gives attention, power and control and is closely connected to how men have learnt to look after themselves emotionally. Men will often enhance their self-esteem through performance and this is where success, achievement and status can become addictive and all-consuming as they have tied this on-going success and growth with their emotional stability.

Within the realm of emotional self-reliance, men have been conditioned to work hard to maintain their mental health. Things get difficult when business success doesn't come or there are problems at work.

Many men are forever fighting off the fear of failure. They fear they have not achieved enough, have not made enough money or they feel compelled and driven to keep busy. The emptiness men often feel can be filled by material objects, substances, sex, or success.

RULE #4 — BE NON-RELATIONAL

\With status being a key man rule, competition becomes a key connector for many men. Typically, men connect with others through active pursuits and hobbies often with a competitive edge. On some levels, there is clearly nothing wrong with this, but it becomes problematic for men when they sustain an injury or are no longer able to compete at a certain level.

I have worked with many men who have suddenly found themselves isolated and depressed because they are no longer able to spend time with their mates as a result of a physical injury. They have struggled because they have not developed the skills or openness to build and sustain fulfilling relationships with their male friends outside of the activity. One of the underlying beliefs men have through this and other rules is that they can only fully rely on themselves. This core survival skill appears to work very well until they hit a crisis point in life and realise their inner resources are not enough.

When it comes to intimate relationships, men often focus on the sexual connection but struggle to put energy and time into developing the emotional connection with their partner.

RULE #5 — HAVE AN OBJECTIFYING ATTITUDE TOWARDS SEXUALITY

Men are often attracted to image, to beauty, and to body. They often ogle or gaze at women. The underlying belief is that women exist to provide pleasure and bodily comfort. When women are turned into sexual objects, sex becomes mechanical and technical, generating the pornography industry and a sexualised culture. With the growth of sex dolls and sex robots, the sexual technical revolution will reach its climax!

Women have been socialised and pressured by the media to dress in certain ways. They do this to fulfil men's notions of women and to titillate men's fantasies. Many women find it uncomfortable aspiring to have the 'perfect' body and wearing the clothes to maintain this. Perhaps we should ask whom and what drives this culture, who owns the fashion houses and who makes money from the lingerie industry. The advertising industry has exaggerated the objectification of women, by portraying certain products as essential, in order for men to be attracted to beautiful women with very little clothes on.

With a focus on the external and objectification, men can often be underdeveloped with regard to their internal skills and expressing the full spectrum of sensuality. When men are focused on the body and on sex, other parts of them are left untapped and unexplored, leaving them experiencing a lack of bodily connection.

RULE #6 — FEAR AND HATE OF HOMOSEXUALITY

Heterosexual men are often extremely vigilant to any suggestion that they are not 'real' men. This includes any suggestion they are not fully heterosexual. They can't abide any hint that they might be gay. This would be seen by many heterosexual men as an attack on their 'real man' status.

Men can be quick to attack a possible slip in machismo, in which the 'pack' keeps up the pretence 'the other' is not like them. Underlying this hatred of homosexuality, can often be a fear of their own inner feelings of insecurity about masculinity.

What we hate or are anxious about in ourselves can often be what we project onto others. In my experience, it is normal for men to question their sexuality and yet it can produce much insecurity. Indeed, I have worked with many men who have 'come out' in the second half of their lives. This is never an easy thing to do. Yet, they feel more confident in their masculinity to be able to embrace their sexuality.

RULE #7 — NORMALISE MALE AGGRESSION

This rule borrows its myth from the 'boys will be boys' discourse, maintaining that boys are naturally aggressive. This view asserts boys and men are violent, due to their hunting and warrior instinct which is needed for the survival of the tribe. This is another rule that is eager to reduce men to one-dimensional beings and culturally it appears we want to perpetuate this rule.

Little boys are taught they should be strong; they need to learn to physically fight and not to allow anyone to push them around. Boys and men are made to protect the 'weaker sex' and need to harness their natural aggression.

Boys and men are expected to train in male skills at every opportunity to make sure they harden up. One such skill is to master the art of banter with quick-draw wit. Humiliating responses are used as a form of self-protection and to prove emotional strength. Banter can be fun but it can also be a passive-aggressive form of communication.

Anger often spills into verbal or physical aggression. It is the one emotion men are 'allowed' to express as it is seen as a strong emotion. Anger has become their default emotion and emotional defence system.

It is part of the 'hard-man' toolbox, but it can also turn inwards with many men exercising anger on themselves, being quick to self-criticise and put themselves down.

PART 3

THE TEN KEYS TO UNDERSTANDING AND UNLOCKING THE INNER LIVES OF MEN

How do men change? Can men change?

Men are often unaware of their emotions and many will deny that emotions have any control over them. They have learnt to keep them well hidden from others and often themselves. This leaves them emotionally isolated.

As humans, we change, grow and develop physically but some of us become emotionally stunted. It appears some people rise to the exciting challenge of change but others find it frightening and remain stuck. What kick starts change? For some of us, it demands a crisis when our old way of doing things no longer works. This crisis can lead people to lean heavier on old coping skills or it can be the wake-up call to try something different.

To make change happen, understanding ourselves is the first step. In the first two parts of this book, I have sought to lay some foundations to how complex change is. The first part explores relationships and our family of origin and how they affect our view of the world and unspoken expectations from ourselves and others. The second part of the book describes a brief history of masculinity and the way it has shaped views and behaviour of men. In this part of the book, we will continue to seek to understand the emotional blocks many men will encounter. For change to happen, understanding will need to be enhanced by emotional connection and hard work.

The ten keys I will describe in this part of the book started as a talk to women entitled '10 tips on how to understand men'. As mentioned in the introduction to this book, if men in relationships are going to change then women will often have to change their expectations of men. Remember Ian from the introduction?

Through therapy, his behaviour was beginning to change and yet his wife struggled to accept the new Ian. She felt as if her role in the relationship and family was being usurped and she struggled to embrace the change. The change in Ian seemed to threaten her and made her feel insecure, almost highlighting her lack of change.

If we want to improve and change our relationships, then when men are ready to change, we as their partners will need to make space for this change to happen.

Emotionally unfit women will typically be flooded by their emotions. Unfit men will typically be in an emotional desert. Women will typically be wet and men will typically be dry. These polarities are both unhealthy and working towards a balance would be much healthier.

The next ten chapters will delve in a little deeper to the secret lives of men and give a few keys on how they can be unlocked. This is really the core of this book.

Each chapter will describe one of the hidden messages about being a man that has constricted his emotions. At the end of each chapter, there will be a toolbox with five keys to unlock the mystery and increase emotional fitness. The five different key levels describe the time and amount of practise needed to implement that tip.

Key one may be an emotional trick and can be implemented immediately and will only take one minute to practise. Key five will take extra work and time and could demand ten minutes or more and will, therefore, demand extra practise.

Change is difficult. If we are going to change, we will need to really desire it, work at it and be disciplined at it.

Let's go!

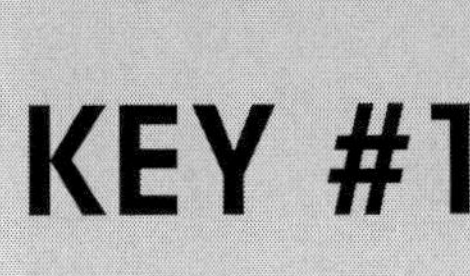

KEY #1

FEELINGS ARE LIKE A FOREIGN LANGUAGE

> 'Men cry. They have tear ducts and lacrimal glands just like other human beings. A man crying is no different from a woman crying. It's natural. Gender roles are toxic when they don't even allow an outlet for pain Cry, men. Cry your heart out.'
>
> — MATT HAIG[23]

'I have no idea what he is thinking', 'He gives nothing away'. I can't recount the number of times that I have heard statements like these from women. The man in their life doesn't talk much, appears to be a mystery and they don't really know him or what is going on inside his head. The truth is that, unfortunately, most men don't really know what is going on inside their heads either. They are often not lying when they say that 'nothing' is going on in there. Unless a problem needs solving, the man's head appears empty.

It appears that for many men they really have no idea what they are thinking or feeling, there really is just nothingness

How was this 'nothingness' developed? The male rules taught men it is emotionally dangerous to reveal too much. They also taught them that the best tool for survival is to hide. Men have learnt to be cool and keep a straight face. Some parents and teachers ask the boy, 'What are you smiling at?' or 'Wipe that smile off your face' and eventually the developing boy learnt to follow the request; the default face, an expressionless mask, or poker face was worn.

In mastering this defence strategy, they have found it difficult to read themselves and have lost touch with their emotions. One important tip to help men deal with the default poker face is to allow their feelings to move their faces. This may mean stretching the face into smiles and other unusual emotional expressions.

Men are quite capable of expressing a full range of feelings, but due to early trauma, gender conditioning and the male code, they have often forgotten this early language. Infant boys are actually more in tune with their feelings than infant girls and typically more empathic. This empathy may be interpreted by parents as demanding or a form of 'neediness'.

Attention from others is perfectly normal and we all need it

As parents, we often want to condition this 'neediness' out of our children through certain techniques. As boys grow and get bigger, parents may reinforce the 'cry-baby' message, followed with 'It's time you grew up'. When boys get a little bigger they may be accused of being attention seekers, which is communicated as annoying behaviour. This reveals a neediness and responses to this like 'stop showing off' or' stop being silly' are received as shaming by boys and men.

Often parents, adults, and professionals can exhibit a derogatory message about attention, when, in fact, it is totally normal and needed. Children and adolescents thrive on attention. If loving, caring attention can be balanced with a healthy sense of growing independence, the child will develop well.

I work with up to fifteen young people a week and one of the most common stories I hear is that they are not getting enough good attention from their parents. Adults, of course, need attention as well but may be a little more sophisticated and subtle in the ways they try to get it.

E-Motions — The body and emotions are one

When an infant feels sad, angry, happy, upset, hungry or lacking attention, they will show this with total full body and verbal expression. Nothing else matters. When they don't feel good, they let you know! They are congruent. They are also naturally empathic; when you smile at them, they can mirror this behaviour.

There is something very natural about infants. This ability to be empathic is also part of their innate survival instinct. If they are crying for something and they aren't given the attention they need, they will eventually learn that this behaviour will not get their needs met. If they hear an angry voice or see an angry face, they will learn this is threatening to their survival. They learn to adjust their behaviour or appease in order to get their needs met. Infants learn they must act in a certain way to please their carers. This is where incongruence begins — the inside world doesn't match their outside world.

As the gap grows between what is felt on the inside and what is revealed on the outside, the harder it is for us to reconcile our own dilemmas. An internal splitting takes place, beginning the process of losing touch with our true selves. Emotions then become disjointed.

Due to early conditioning and the male code, boys lose an ability to express their emotions. This is not helped by a reduced vocabulary. Boys typically suffer from alexithymia. By the age of seven, boys have learnt to shut down and are unwilling to express their feelings in public places, afraid of being shamed or humiliated.

By the age of ten, boys learn there are geographically accepted places where they are allowed to express a broader range of feelings. These may include team sports, music, and acting. Engaging with animals has also proved to be a way in which boys can express their tender and vulnerable feelings safely. Since owning our own dog, it has been amazing to see how often my boys want to be close to her. They want to cuddle her, be cuddled by her, show their love and affection through communication and express their empathy and affection in a completely natural uninhibited way.

THE THEATRE OF FREE, UNINHIBITED EMOTIONAL EXPRESSION

Sport increasingly plays a major part in the lives of boys and men. It creates a magical theatre for 'shameless' free expression of emotion. Culturally, sport has sanctioned a male's expression of the full spectrum of emotions, with no risk to their masculine identity. Team contact sports, such as football and rugby, can create a tribal atmosphere and pack out arenas where men can satisfy full emotional expression.

Equally, when men play football, the full spectrum of emotions can be displayed freely, uninhibited and without risk of embarrassment. In this arena, which is generally male populated and male-dominated, men appear to fully enjoy their togetherness. This 'tribal' environment can produce a sort of spiritual connection, in which men enjoy the power of their voices in song and chant. Of course, there is the darker side of violence lurking within these tribal events, which reveals itself in the mob, the gangs and the violence on and off the pitch.

GOAL!

When a 'goal' is scored, the male follower expresses uninhibited joy and delight. The ecstatic scenes of England's journey in the 2018 football World Cup bear witness to this. Men expressed joy, perhaps even more than they had when their wife or partner gave birth to a son or daughter. In the moment of free expression, men can be seen jumping with joy, crying tears of joy or sadness, displaying nail-biting and real anxiety and, of course, lots of aggression.

On the field, once a goal is scored, the sportsmen will enjoy a big display of extroverted emotion, including massive smiles, dancing, somersaults, hugging and kissing and nobody in the arena will raise an eyebrow. This behaviour is seen as totally acceptable when the all-important goal is scored.

There will be many hardened men watching this 'feminine' display of affection and no one will accuse them of being 'gay' or 'pussies'

Soon though, there is an emotional and physical shutdown. The men leave the stadium and return to the default position of muteness, with a poker face and emotional restriction. When observing the supporters leaving the arena, it can sometimes be very difficult to identify whether their team has won or lost, as the men return to their normal default state.

EMOTIONAL RELEASE: ALCOHOL, DRUGS AND SEX.

Male addiction to alcohol, substances, and sex has reached epidemic proportions in many countries all over the world. Both men and women use and abuse alcohol as a way of loosening themselves up in social situations. It helps them to relax.

When slightly (or heavily) inebriated, men can express a wider range of feelings and say things to other men that they may not say when not under the influence. 'I love you mate' can be said without fear or worry. It would very rarely be said without the loosening effect of alcohol. Some men may find themselves crying and revealing more vulnerable and tender feelings and, of course, alcohol can be the tap to release unhealthy anger or violent rage.

Later on in the book, we will explore in more detail the link between men's need for sex and emotional expression. My feeling is that if men were more in tune with the full expression of their emotions then they would be more sensual, tender, and emotionally empathic.

A healthy sex drive is, of course, a joyous and beautiful part of humanity. But when one is driven by it and it becomes a sole expression of many emotions, then it is time to take note. Pornography has become pervasive in society and filters into many areas of life producing a clinical and mechanical view of sexuality, often reducing sex to grunts, groans, groins, genitals, and the passing of fluids.

MEN HAVE JUST SIX WORDS TO EXPRESS THE FULL RANGE OF EMOTIONS

I rarely ask men how they feel. It feels pointless. Many men have a very limited emotional vocabulary. Many will say 'I don't know' or 'I am not sure what you mean', almost like I am speaking a foreign language. Often, men will look extremely uncomfortable or awkward and usually avoid the question by returning to a cognitive position or rational discussion. If I do ask them, I can guarantee they will say one of the following phrases:

1. Alright
2. Not bad
3. Good
4. Fine
5. Okay
6. Normal

JUST BE 'NORMAL'

None of the words or phrases listed above describe in any accuracy an emotional state. In the world of emotions, these six words or phrases would reside in the happy/content quadrant. When people are emotionally fit, they are able to access all of their emotions and express the right emotion at the right time. Men have been trained as boys to always be 'alright'. They learn not to cry and to not expect comfort, reassurance or tenderness. They have learnt they have to rely on themselves and others expect them to always be alright, good etc.

This theory is never more evident than when boys and men tell me they are feeling 'normal'. Normal is, however, not an emotion. They are describing their feeling state as stable. It is, to them, a familiar place. It is a similar state to most other boys and men, a sort of placid neutrality where they don't feel too much and are not too bothered by dismay or elation.

For a man, feeling 'normal' suggests the man thinks he is fitting in. Identifying as 'normal' would also highlight the man's limited awareness of his feeling state and limited vocabulary. One of the reasons why they want to be seen as 'normal' is that they are terrified of being exposed, of standing out, of being different.

Many men only have two emotional settings, normal and abnormal. Abnormal feelings will include uncomfortable feelings such as sadness, anxiety, hurt and shame. These feelings will make him hot under the collar. Typically, for many men this abnormal state will be expressed as anger.

DECLARING A WAR ON TERROR

Boys have learnt to feel pain but not express it. This terrifying message cripples boys and men emotionally. They learn that revealing their inner feelings is dangerous — they risk being seen as a woman and less of a man. They learn that 'real men don't do feelings'. Men are in fear they might in some way be exposed, experience shame and feel less than they should. This is the war on terror I want to wage.

The terror of the internal world has led men to externalise these feelings and create monster emotions which is well depicted through the Marvel character of the 'Incredible Hulk'. Dr Bruce Banner, who as a small man sometimes feels angry. The emotion overwhelms him and turns him into a frightening monster who completely takes over the human. The Hulk is a great example of how men fail to express the right emotion at the right time. When one emotion feeds into the others, it can turn into a monster.

EMOTIONAL EJACULATION

When a nation or man feels terrified, they often unleash their internal terror onto others. The surge of pain (anger, fear, resentment) they feel inside is often allowed to build up, until they can no longer hold it in, and it explodes into the world. It is like an emotional ejaculation. The 'war on terror' I want to wage is to enable boys and men to take responsibility for their feelings and to normalise the expression of the whole spectrum of emotion. This could bring real healing into the world.

I want to unleash a war on the man rules, a war on societal and gender conditioning and a war on the myth that there is only one way of being a man. I want to wage a war on the internal terror that many men feel and invite them to allow their frightening feelings and fears to transform them.

For the rest of this chapter, I want to help you understand what the man may be thinking and feeling. I also want to offer some tips on how to move from emotional muteness to emotional fitness. Indeed, the muteness appears to be at the heart of the problem and I have named it 'the trauma of emotional restriction'. This trauma leaves many men struggling to understand themselves and their feelings.

It may be linked to why men are more commonly on the autistic spectrum than women. The emotional brain is underdeveloped and crucial parts of it are left unwired, due to the reasons I have mentioned above. Please note, I am aware of the complexity of autism and do not wish to minimise this condition. Indeed, some would see it as a superpower!

I have worked with hundreds of men and boys individually and in groups during the past twenty years. This understanding has been confirmed over and over again. With the right support, men have been able to develop their emotional fitness, become more emotionally expressive, and feel more alive. When men begin to understand the internal working of the typical man, using the tools provided below, then I believe in the majority of cases emotional fitness can be increased.

HEALTHY EMOTIONAL EXPRESSION

All of us have the capacity to express the whole spectrum of emotions. To explain healthy emotional expression, I often use the 'Feeling grid' (See below). Emotionally fit people have the capacity to access and express the right feeling at the right time. In the grid below, there are four basic feelings (and clearly there are many more) but this tool is a good starting point.

We all have the possibility of feeling hundreds of different feelings every day, but we may only be aware of a few. It is possible to be firmly planted in one of the grid quadrants or to experience a fusion of the feelings. Right now as I write, I am conscious of being tired, slightly irritated, anxious, and a little sad. Just by noticing this and grounding the feeling with an experience or event is sometimes enough for the feeling to disperse.

When we are more aware of our feelings, we have more chance of responding to them and controlling their expression. Each feeling should be acknowledged and felt. When we can do this, we have a greater possibility of being fully connected. For example, at any time of day, a feeling could be triggered through an unconscious connection.

A sad feeling connected to my father could pop into my head right now. If I ignore it, then it could linger or be suppressed. If we keep ignoring feelings, eventually they morph into an unknown mass often stored in the body and we have essentially lost control of that feeling. But if I acknowledge it and feel it, then it can be dispersed.

All a feeling wants from you is to be felt, once it is felt it can disperse. If the right feeling is not felt, then it gets stuck and will demand attention

---

Feelings are not our enemies. They are our friends. When felt, they can keep us in a healthy and balanced state. Many of us have lost touch with our senses and have forgotten the importance of trusting our senses. Common sense is in short supply in the modern world. Taste has been reduced to blandness, hearing reduced to white noise, sight to looking at screens. Touch is too dangerous. Feeling and our intuitive sense, has often been replaced by its rational cousin — thinking.

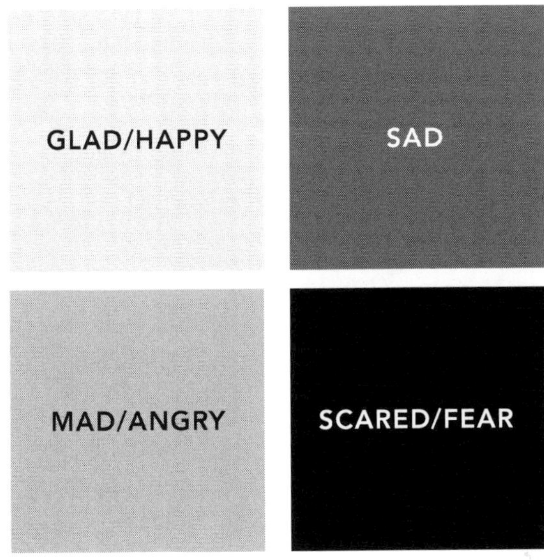

When we feel the right feeling at the right time the 'grid' will remain quite uniformed and we stay grounded and connected. On some occasions, one quadrant could become larger when a feeling demands more attention. This is absolutely normal and understandable and will resume its typical size once the feeling has been felt and processed. This would be the case during a traumatic episode, bereavement, or any other event that generates a strong response.

I work with many clients who were told that to cry was to show weakness and the result is they bottle up their emotion. It then comes out in unhealthy ways (such as anger) or it seeps out through the body. If we don't allow sadness to flow and try and dam it up, the dam will eventually break. There will then be a flood of emotions which could cause all sorts of damage.

THE EMOTIONAL GYM

It is no surprise the majority of men have flabby emotional muscles. These are in desperate need of toning. Most of us are familiar with the importance of physical exercise and the discipline it takes to build core strength and to develop muscle. Many men will watch what they eat and be aware of the importance of eating a healthy and balanced diet.

Exercise your emotional muscles

However, few men invest time, energy, commitment, and money into developing their emotional muscles. Many consider it to be a waste of time and money seeing an emotional fitness coach, counsellor or psychotherapist. They will not consider entering an emotional gym to exercise their emotions and probably feel they have their emotions under control. In my practice, men will complete an intensive therapeutic workout, dealing with present issues and then sign up for regular emotion gym sessions.

These clients describe feeling the same 'buzz' at the end of the session as they would after a physical workout. Emotions have shifted. There is a new sense of entering into the world of emotion. The men who go through this process feel challenged and strengthened. They leave feeling fresher, lighter, and at one with themselves.

MEN'S DEFAULT EMOTIONAL GRID

When the emotional spectrum is reduced due to the male rules, social conditioning and emotional restraint a typical man's emotional grid may look more like the feeling grid pictured below. Having been taught to feed one emotion over all the others, many men have reduced their ability in expressing other feelings and then lose the ability to express them freely and at the right time. This default grid has become normal for him.

It is like a man going to a gym and just toning his right biceps. This muscle will become pronounced and strong but will leave the rest of his body flabby and weak. Most men have over-worked the emotional muscle of anger so it has become dominant and left little space for other emotional muscles to develop.

When in this state, he has reduced his skills at expressing other feelings and the only place for them to go is inside. They are then left to fester and build and are at risk of seeping out through the different states of anger creating greater risk of being out of control. When a person's emotional grid has become out of sync, the other emotions are reduced and muted. This reduction can also prevent men from fully expressing other parts of themselves.

When a boy has been conditioned to be hard and tough then his tender part is reduced. When he is told to not be a wuss or to fear anything then he loses touch with his ability to access appropriate risk. When he has been told big boys don't cry, his ability to be with his sadness has been reduced. At this point, parts of himself have been locked up waiting to be discovered.

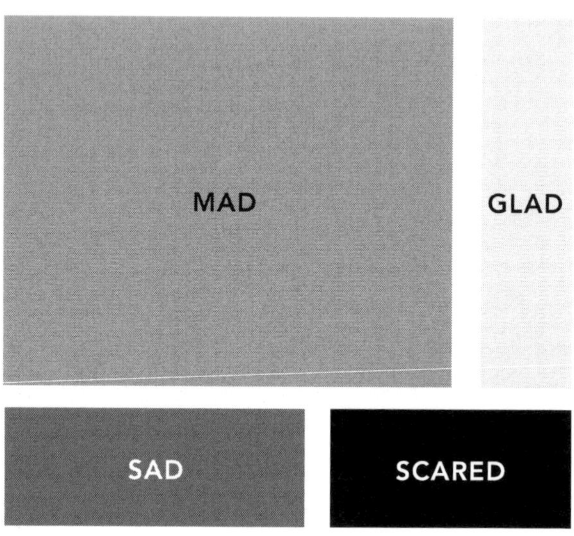

Typically, girls and women have been told not to be angry and so their ability to access healthy anger has been reduced. They have been told it's alright to cry and so their sad quadrant may have become dominant. For another person, their scared quarter may be enlarged as their threat sensor gets stuck on. They then view the world mainly through this emotion triggered by a past experience.

THE MACHINE IS BROKEN — GO TO THE GARAGE FOR HELP

Many male clients may arrive at the first session expecting to be treated like a car going in for its service or a MOT. Men can sometimes tend to think that their minds and mental health are like machines and it's only when they are broken or don't perform as well that they give them some attention.

'If it isn't broken, then don't fix it' is often a man's mantra

---

If signs of wear begin to show, the first course of action is often to blame others. The second course of action is band-aid where they may try and change and do things differently. Usually, they are unable to sustain it and the underlying problem remains unaddressed. Usually, by the time men come for counselling, they are in crisis and losing control of their relationship, business, and life.

For many of these men, it is apparent they want me to fix them. It is almost as if they are saying, 'okay, my machine/car is broken and my mechanical skills are exhausted and I now have to take it to the professional garage'. This is for many men a huge and courageous step, often inducing shame and vulnerability.

They can be quick to apologise for wasting my time and recommend I do a little tinkering to sort them out and ultimately fix them. It is as if they want me to change the oil and the brake pads, sort out the malfunction, and get them back on the road again. When I meet a male client like this, they are ultimately scared as they realise something is wrong, that they can no longer hide it and they are desperate for me to work my magic and sort them out.

It is in these moments I can almost visibly see the little boy, the fearful little boy who has been trying so hard all his life to 'play the game' to get it right and to keep others happy. I am acutely aware of his sense of feeling exposed, his neediness, and his longing to be looked after.

Of course, I see my job and role as one who can assist and create the right environment for growth and change to happen and I want to do whatever I can to help. I have tried complying with these men by being the advice-giver; the mechanic; or the caring, all-knowing parent. Let me say it clearly — IT DOESN'T WORK!!

My message therefore to these men is this, 'I cannot fix you!'

Darren finally plucked up the courage to come to counselling. He was losing control of his emotions and his tears just kept bursting out. During our first session, he shared how scared he was and how much pressure he had in his head. Darren found himself bursting into tears for much of the session as he shared his story, his shame and what he had been doing for the first half of his life. He talked about how the boy part of him has dominated him and he appeared to be stuck in the boy.

A week later, Darren was in his second session and he reported that he had noticed things had changed. He realised that for one of the first times in his life, he had begun to take responsibility for his feelings. He was becoming more aware of his expectations of others and the way he treated them. He cried more during this session and was becoming much more aware of his feelings. Nearing the end of this session, Darren said this,

> *'I came here wanting to be fixed, but I now realise with your help I need to fix myself'.*

Darren had got the essence of the work and of growth really quickly and was on his way to moving from the boy to the man.

Likewise, near the end of a first session with a new client, Billy, he asked me if I could help him and my reply was 'No'. This clearly took him aback and he replied with, 'Oh, that's really disappointing'. During the session, he had told me how he has been suffering from depression for many years and had received advice and help from many different therapists across different disciplines.

Along with medication and input, Billy had stabilised in many ways. I clarified my 'no' by saying, that I didn't have 'the power to fix' him. I did, however, say, I could create the right environment for him to help himself. I told Billy he was the expert on himself and that for change to happen he would need to trust himself. He got this and understood the process of actualisation.

Billy completed two further sessions and returned for an MOT about two months later. He seemed to be in more control and content and was able to manage his emotions much better. After that session, Billy didn't book any further sessions and I think he had finally taken responsibility for his emotional development. I ultimately feel there are no short cuts to growth; it will take challenge, hard work and discipline.

Both Darren and Billy got this but for some clients who hear that I can't fix them or notice my resistance to giving them some quick advice, this may leave them feeling dismayed. This has been what they had hoped for and what they had expected within their traditional survival strategies and so shatters their assumptions.

I haven't just conjured this view up. This is not just a bullish, make them feel the pain approach. This understanding has come out of experience of working with many men and therefore knowing this approach does not work. The only way men can actually change internally is to be prepared to do some hard inner work, to learn to take responsibility for their behaviour, their emotions, and for their language.

Unfortunately, not all clients leave their final sessions in that way. I have had some leave angry and dissatisfied. Others leave with a sense of feeling it has not worked and I did not help them.

To be prepared to begin an emotional gym programme to tone up some flabby emotional muscles, expect to endure some emotional stretching. In my view, when it comes to emotional growth and developing emotional muscles, there really is no emotional gain without feeling emotional pain.

SHORT EMOTIONAL FITNESS PROGRAMME

Becoming emotionally fit, like being physically fit, requires time, hard work and has to be practised and rehearsed. To tone up flabby emotional muscles men will need to join an emotional or mental gym where they can regularly stretch, flex and build emotional muscles. Many men have not become aware of the need to develop their emotional life and remain stuck in a developmental time warp.

Some men have put a lot of emotion into anger: their 'angry muscle' is bulging whereas other emotional muscles relating to tenderness, vulnerability, pain or sadness may be severely underdeveloped. If this happens (and it often does), it will cause pain to emerge in other areas of their lives. When one emotion has become dominant, it is easy for men to lose touch with other parts of themselves and to become one dimensional.

Many women have been given an advantage in the expression of a range of emotions due to gender conditioning. But like any skill or talent, one has to keep practising to continue to grow in this area. Some women are not emotionally fit, they may have accommodated a default emotion which has become unhealthy.

Women may have a broader emotional vocabulary and a greater ability to express the right feeling, but like any form of fitness we have to keep training and learn about unfamiliar muscles to have a balanced all-round fitness. So, this system is for women as well as men and may even be a good programme to do together with your partner in order to develop relational fitness.

When I work with men to increase their emotional fitness, I use my five-stage model called **A.W.A.R.E.** which describes the five different components to increasing and developing emotional fitness. At the end of each stage, there will be some specific tools to increase emotional fitness.

1. **A**TTENTION — 'Give attention to your tension'

Emotions are information and when we give attention to our body and tensions we become more emotionally fit. Emotionally fit people are awake to their bodily sensations, they are attuned to any changes and able to respond and listen to what the body is saying.

The majority of men have lost touch with their body and ultimately with their senses and have learnt to spend the majority of the time in their heads.

Often men's bodies are treated as machines and men spend their time building, beating and working their bodies. Few men listen to their bodies

---

Men have often not learnt to listen to their bodies, to pay attention to the aches, strains and pains. They have struggled to identify the e-motion emoted through motion. This has often left them out of sync and instead of expressing their emotion they have suppressed them and left their bodies to carry them and hold them.

This can have serious consequences on physical health. When men learn to listen to their bodies, they can learn to identify their emotions easier and allow the body to inform them of an emotion rather than ignoring or resetting the 'everything is normal' button.

Your body and emotions are at one and are in E-motion together

The 'pain in the neck', headache, shoulder tension, teeth grinding, chest tightness, clenched fists, lightness in the stomach are all indicators and clues to an emotional state of being. The nagging groin pain, drooping shoulders, and emerging grin are all bodily tips in helping us embrace the emotion in that moment. When we start to tune in to these emotions rather than tune them out and increasingly becoming aware of them, then we can feel the right emotion at the right time and become more congruent.

The male poker face has limited facial expression. Often, we will have a default face. I discovered my default face or resting face while looking in my car rearview mirror. I was suddenly made aware of the face I offer to the world and it wasn't a pleasant sight. I now practise smiling more and am aware of my relaxed poker face much more often. We need to practise moving our face.

TOOLBOX TO INCREASE ATTENTION

- **FACE IT** — find your default face when you look in the rear-view mirror in your car, sit with that for a while — what does your face present to the world? Practise moving your face more to unstick the 'poker face' — try smiling and expressing other emotions — watch for others' reactions. Check your face in the mirror throughout the day — does your face match your feelings inside?

- **BODY SCAN** — listen to your bodily sensations and have regular body scans or check-ins throughout the day. What is your body telling you? When you are aware of a tension, give it some attention. Remember — emotions are information.

2. **W**ORD BANK

As mentioned earlier, most men do not have a broad emotional vocabulary and many are suffering from alexithymia — 'without words for emotions'. Before a man can become more emotionally expressive, he may need to literally expand his vocabulary. Emotional language may literally feel like a foreign language. He may have learnt a few classic phrases or words to get through but is soon floundering for language.

Often, men can become stuck in social and relational situations, because they have a reduced ability to express what they feel. They may also resort to staying in the rational part of themselvcs and hide behind their 'facts' instead of engaging in discussion. During an argument, when the other expresses that they do not understand them, they may just resort to speaking louder and slower — **LET ME REPEAT MYSELF AGAIN** (the Englishman abroad approach), but this doesn't help.

When men do this, they are convinced they are making perfect sense and the fault is with the other. Men may then feel that the other person is deliberately 'doing their head in' and just 'messing' with them. This feeling is almost always a shame-based reaction.

When a man is in this situation, here is an approach which might help. This will also build shame resilience. When a person complains that they did not understand what you said, ask them which part of what you just said they did not understand. This will help to avoid repeating yourself word for word.

TOOLBOX TO DEVELOP EMOTIONAL VOCABULARY

1. **Learn more words.** In developing your emotional word bank, try sitting down with the feeling grid each day for two minutes. Write down different words you have felt during the day and expand your word bank. You could also use the 'feeling wheel' (see below). Take three words a day and try and use them throughout the day. Having a greater command of a broader vocabulary can prevent conflict occurring over relatively small issues.

2. **Put a name to the feeling.** When we can name a feeling, it can quickly help us disperse the feeling. Naming the right feeling immediately helps us to relax. Equally, acknowledging the feeling internally can allow that feeling to disperse. Often, all a feeling needs is to be acknowledged, accepted and expressed.

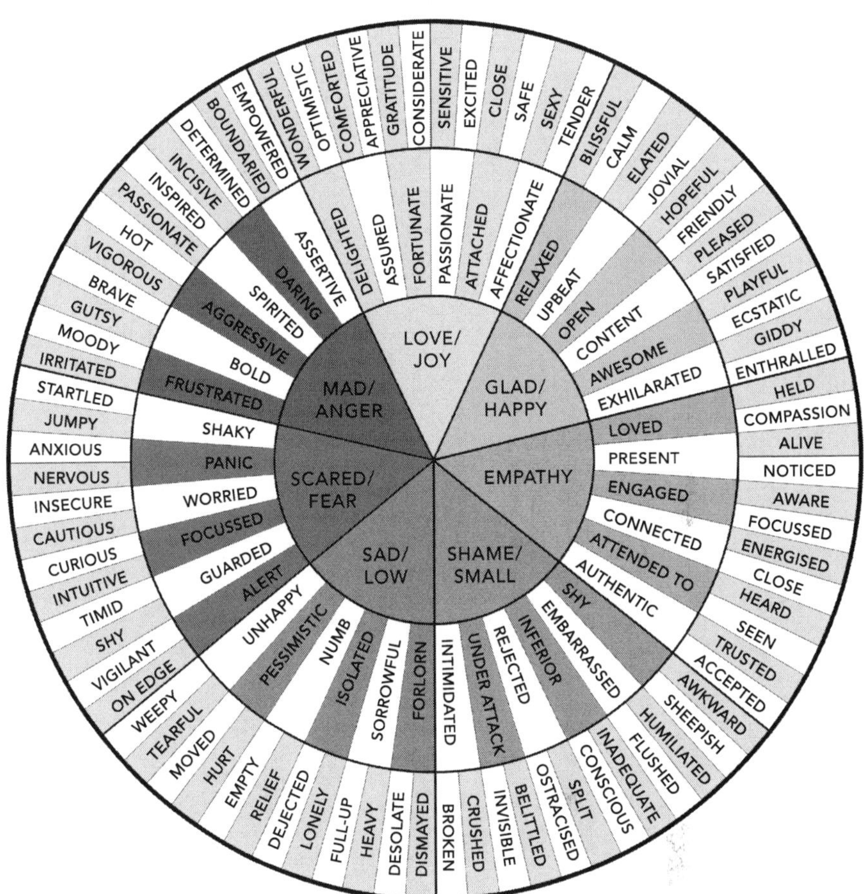

3. **A**CCEPT YOUR FEELINGS

We often find it hard to accept our feelings. Many of us use a huge amount of energy and time ignoring and avoiding uncomfortable emotions. One of the most difficult things to do in life is to feel our feelings, especially the painful ones such as anger, despair, envy, sadness, shame, and fear. These are often referred to as 'negative' feelings.

As we become more aware of the fuller spectrum of emotions, it will be made clear that we have spent much energy, time, and money on depressing, uncomfortable feelings and doing all we can to avoid those feelings. When we find the courage to face the difficult feelings and to embrace the right feeling at the right time, we have a greater possibility of being congruent and who we are in that moment. This stage appears quite simple but is the most difficult.

Feelings are neither positive nor negative, they just are

Clive came to my practice struggling with depression, motivation and lack of energy. It was not long before he was talking about how he disliked himself, compared himself to others and was trying to live up to his parents' expectations. Clive told me how he felt deeply angry and unhappy. He spoke of how he was disgusted with himself, felt ashamed of who he was, and how he had been hiding parts of himself he found hard to accept. He had surrounded himself with fixers and was stuck in an emotionally immature place.

He expressed these difficult feelings and began to accept the truth of them in relation to his life. This is a really difficult process as many of us have been told to be positive, suck it up and never mention your truth. As I listened to Clive, I became aware of the lights turning on and that he was beginning to 'wake up' to this new way of seeing things. Clive's work had begun. He started to accept his feelings and had begun to have the courage to be who he is.

Emotional fitness means this:

Express the right feelings, at the right time, in the right way.

When we fail to do this and ignore, avoid, suppress, or project our feelings, we are psychologically self-harming. Remember all a feeling requires is to be felt. Once the right feeling is felt and acknowledged internally or externally, then it can disperse. If we fail to do this, a feeling will get stuck and cling onto us. When this happens, we lose connection with it and are in danger of losing control of that feeling. They can end up clogging up our body and head or morphing into a different feeling.

TOOLBOX TO INCREASE YOUR ACCEPTANCE OF YOUR FEELINGS

- There are no negative emotions. Remember the mantra: 'No one can make me feel anything'.
- Start saying — 'I feel' rather than, 'I think'.

4. **R**ELEASE. TAKE RESPONSIBILITY FOR YOUR FEELINGS. DEVELOP EMOTIONAL REGULATION

The fourth stage of the emotional fitness programme is to practise releasing emotion. So far within this programme, you will have practised attending to your feelings and being aware of bodily sensations. Your word bank will be in 'credit' and you will be seeking to accept all feelings as friends that will enhance your life. These steps are all important because they will help you become more in control of your emotions and make them more regulated. This next step is about learning to release the right emotion at the right time, which will allow it to fully disperse.

The first part of this process is to fully take responsibility for your emotional expression. Most of us react but we can learn to respond. When we are emotionally fit, we have the choice in how we express our emotions. Ultimately, this will give us the ability to regulate our emotional response.

We have two choices on how to exercise our feelings, we can 'inspress' or 'express'. When we 'inspress', we acknowledge the feeling inside. When we express, we allow it to be spoken or moved externally, so the feeling becomes as 'visible' as possible using our expanded vocabulary to give the feeling a depth and a shape. The closer we get to this expression, the more fit we will be with the benefit of being congruent.

When we are congruent, our interior and exterior worlds match each other. There is no longer any split between the two. This is a much healthier place to be; the phrase 'what you see is what you get' describes a product we trust but also a person who is congruent, who doesn't conceal something. Ideally, this is where the emotionally 'rounded' person is heading.

When the goal is scored, the delay between the ball hitting the back of the net and the expression of pure, unhindered joy is minimal — this is what congruence looks like

---

I have learnt to express myself when I am anxious and often do this when I am going to address a large group of people. I generally like public speaking and embrace a healthy anxiety to give me the spark and energy to deliver a talk with some passion. Before the talk, I will often naturally be anxious. I will be conscious of this and release this through internally acknowledging this to myself — an 'inspress'.

When I begin my talk, I sometimes feel overly anxious and may notice parts of my body shaking or my mouth feeling dry. I will then express to the audience that I am aware of the feeling of anxiety. To be honest, many of the audience will already have noticed this, so I am stating the obvious.

After I have expressed my anxiety, it disperses. I see the audience relax and I immediately feel more relaxed and in the moment.

Another example is when a person patronises you. You have a choice of either ignoring the sensations and holding the anger inside, reacting to the comment with a passive-aggressive response or responding to how you felt when you heard what they said. The response may sound something like 'Please don't belittle me.' When we are able to feel the right feelings at the right time, the feeling will not need to linger or stick to us, it can pass and leave us lighter.

Growth in emotional expression is recognised when we lessen the time between the event and the emotional expression. Some of the learning at this stage is about reviewing and reflecting on events and practising how we could have dealt with that situation better or rehearsing how we could have responded better or more authentically.

Emotions are fluid. They need to move and flow. Sometimes they are very strong and may rise up suddenly. At other times, they will be much more placid. When we experience a very difficult event, such as the death of a loved one, our default emotional grid may be flooded with sadness. Working through the grief will be difficult and the flow of emotion may be stuck for a while. Sadness is asking for time: it wants to be deeply felt and it's not in a rush to move. It is important to acknowledge this and stay in the lagoon for a period.

At the right time, the beauty of sadness will nudge you to move on. It will be our emotional awareness that will allow us to hear and feel this nudge and allow our self to let go. Gradually, our emotional grid will return to a healthy, normal state, with the ability to feel a broader range of emotions. We will be able to respond to those feelings in a healthier, mature way.

TOOLBOX TO AID EMOTIONAL EXPRESSION

- Practise staying with the feeling as it arises. Don't be quick to move it, avoid it or project it but respect and listen to it.
- Remember that you have a choice in how to exercise your emotion. You can react or you can respond. Practise inspressing and expressing on different occasions.

5. **E**MPATHY FOR SELF — LISTEN TO YOURSELF AND LOVE YOURSELF

Empathy literally means to 'walk in the shoes of another'. When we are empathic, we seek to understand and feel what it is like being that other person. This final step of the emotional fitness programme is crucial as it will help you to maintain your fitness as you build emotional resilience.

Empathy for self is ultimately getting into your own head and having self-compassion for yourself by connecting to your inner feelings and letting yourself off the hook. Internally, there is a constant chatter or inner dialogue, in which we are ultimately listening and talking to ourselves.

Some believe that people who talk to themselves are going mad. I think this is nonsense and actually, the people who are not aware of their inner dialogue are at risk of generating split personalities. I often talk out loud to myself, just to make sure I can hear what I am saying. I will concede that talking out loud to yourself in the company of others can be a little embarrassing but nothing more.

For many of us, our inner chatter is of the negative variety where we are telling ourselves off for being stupid, an idiot, or useless. We essentially spend time beating ourselves up, putting ourselves down and punishing ourselves with the constant refrains of 'should', 'must', 'could' and 'ought'.

Self-empathy is the discipline part of the fitness where we have to will ourselves out of bed in the morning to stick to our routine. Self-empathy will require us to identify and capture the negative self-talk and replace it with compassionate words to ourselves. This is literally about being kind to ourselves and refusing to beat ourselves up. When we get practised in this self-soothing skill we prevent ourselves remaining on the cycle of shame, we feel more positive and we build emotional resilience.

TOOLBOX TO LEARN SELF-EMPATHY

- Practise listening to your inner chatter and say kind things to yourself
- Capture the negative words/discourse you constantly tell yourself

If you practise the tools from the **AWARE** emotionally fit system, I am confident you will increase your emotional fitness. Below, I have left you with a few more tips and tools to help you on your way. Go for it!

EMOTIONAL FITNESS TOOLBOX

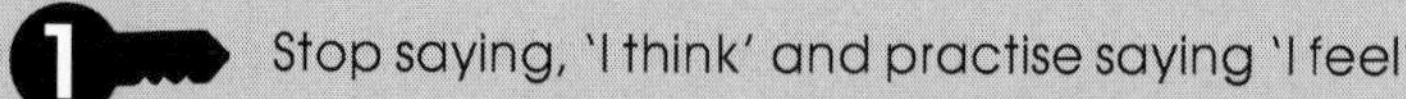

1. Stop saying, 'I think' and practise saying 'I feel'

2. Work on relational emotional fitness by spending time together. I often suggest to couples that they could do the 9-minute exercise. One person talks for three minutes and the other listens. If there is silence within the three minutes, then stay with the silence. Then swap. The final three minutes is for mutual feedback. Extend this practise by doing fifteen or twenty-one minutes.

3. Create a safe space to check in. When we refitted our bathroom, my wife and I bought an extra-large bath. Part of our practise every week is to share a bath and spend time 'talking in the tub' (tub time). This works out to be a great little container where we sometimes thrash out difficult things and try and resolve them in the tub before we get out. Regularly check in with yourself, partner, and friends.

4. Children, dogs, and working in groups are great for developing emotional fitness.

5. Work on all the tools highlighted in **AWARE**

KEY #2

MEN OFTEN FEEL THE NEED TO CONSTANTLY PROVE THEIR MASCULINITY

'The three most destructive words that every man receives when he's a boy is when he's told to 'be a man.''

— JOE EHRMANN, COACH AND FORMER NFL PLAYER[24]

Men learn early on in their lives that masculinity is a slippery state and to belong to 'the club' one has to remain vigilant and alert. The majority of men would never consider this pressure but subconsciously they know it exists and will do almost anything to maintain their status. One of the tools that society and most cultures use to keep men playing by the rules is the 'real man' discourse. The construction of the 'Real Man' discourse is rooted in a hierarchical view of masculinity. This enforces a competitive environment shoring up an immature and insecure masculinity.

Often men feel a fear they will not measure up and that as a result they could be rejected from the male club, relegated to the second division and at risk of being an outcast. Boys and men will regularly hear the refrain that they need to 'step up!' The fear leaves men constantly assessing their status within the hierarchy and in some way accepting this position.

Boys and men will have worked out the 'pecking order' and who the 'top dog',' alpha male', 'hardest' or 'cool' guys are. The rest of the group will sort themselves into their positions of nerds, geeks, wimps, and losers. I have heard this clearly articulated by boys in the schools I work in. The most problematic position for many boys is not knowing which group they belong to or not being able to associate with a group.

The constant fear driving the 'real man' discourse is that a man will be seen as soft and feminine. The higher a man can reach in the hierarchy protected by position and power, the fewer questions and accusations will be made against his fragile status. Men will do all they can to avoid being called a wuss, wet, pussy, soft, small, moist or anything else that might link them to the feminine and female genitalia.

THE MESSAGES MEN HEAR

Proving your 'manhood' is linked to the 'man rules' which has been reinforced by the real man discourse. Being biologically male is not enough to be a man as you have to fulfil a list of conditions. At the root of the 'real man' discourse is the fear that it's not enough to be biologically male, you have to prove which gender you belong to. The following phrases are the ammunition commonly used.

BE A MAN! — This phrase implies there is one way of displaying masculinity. To comply with this, one must essentially know or find out what being a man means.

MAN-UP! — A common term that ultimately means toughen up, be strong, be resilient and show no vulnerability. I have even heard women say this to other women. Often parents can be heard saying this to their children.

ARE YOU MAN ENOUGH? — The challenge of having enough of 'man' within. Are you able to do what needs to be done and what real men should do?

WHAT SORT OF MAN ARE YOU? — This challenging question implies your status of masculinity is under threat, because someone is confused about why you are not acting according to expectations.

CALL YOURSELF A MAN! — Similar to the above statement. The questioner is confused by your actions and feels there must be a mistake. Can you be sure you belong to that gender group?

WHAT ARE YOU, MAN OR MOUSE? — Real men are big, hard and tough but you are acting like a small, scared, soft mammal.

GROW SOME BALLS! — A direct hit on male genitalia which is always painful! The very place men may actually hold their softness, vulnerability, and tenderness is under attack. Real men will have 'balls of steel' or 'big balls' that will reveal their ultimate toughness.

WHAT A PATHETIC EXCUSE FOR A MAN — A full frontal shame attack insulting the man for even trying to be part of that gender group and making sure he is unworthy to actually be a man.

YOU'RE ACTING LIKE A GIRL — Also can include 'stop being a girl' and one-word insults mentioned above. You are acting like the 'weaker, emotional sex' - the other gender - and to be a man you can't associate or show similar traits. When this phrase is used, it is obviously a sexist attack and demeaning to girls, women, boys, and men.

CRYING LIKE A BABY! — May also include 'crying like a girl' and 'It's enough to make a grown man cry'. The message is clear: if men express sadness through moisture, they will be accused of 'blubbering like a child' or be associated with being a woman. Real men should not allow their eyes to sweat and instead, work hard for their tear ducts to dry up!

The messages about the 'right' kind of man to be are being reinforced through peers and media. The messages men receive can also be somewhat confusing and can appear contradictory. Examples of this can regularly be found in magazines which target men. According to these popular magazines, real men should do the following four things to make themselves feel big:

- **Eat Beef** — the magazine says this will help the men to build strength and power. No soft veggies allowed!

- **Build brawn/body** — the 'beefy bodies' with well-toned six-pack and plenty of muscle on display. Be hard, rigid and impenetrable.
- **Breasts**/body — enjoy looking at women's breasts, make lewd comments whenever possible, and sneak a crafty peek at cleavage as often as you can. Have sex as much as possible, fulfilling the old conquest mentality and have sex in as many positions as possible.
- **Booze** — drink copious amount of **beer** — real men should be able to hold their drink and hold a pint glass at all times.

> 'Women can't be too thin, men can't be too hard.'
>
> —TERRENCE REAL[25]

ARE YOU A REAL MAN OR A FAKE MAN?

Faking it until you make it is perhaps the only way many boys and men get through the tough years of proving their manhood. At these tender stages in life, it is all about survival. Some men have the courage of 'coming out' of the faking stage, while others are caught in the trap of the 'real man' game.

The 'real' man concept is a constant source of shame for men. The fake men have to achieve a benchmark, pass a test and fulfil certain criteria to be considered 'proper' or 'real' men. It is not enough to just be biologically male — you must be a REAL man. This has been a constant theme in the world of 'Marvel' where men are 'super' and 'iron'. When men conform to the real man status in 'real' life they will be known as heroes, this includes men who go to war or who do extraordinary feats. These norms shore up hegemonic masculinity (dominant expression of masculinity) and stereotyping. It prevents an exploration of different masculinities and creates a mono-cultural accepted way of being a man.

If as a man you fail to come up to these markers then you are reduced to less of a man, not real, not good enough and left in a constant state of insecurity, left to prove your manhood. Even when men consider themselves to have reached the benchmark it can so easily slip away. Belonging to the 'real man' club can absorb a considerable amount of time and emotional energy.

LESSONS ABOUT REAL FROM THE VELVETEEN RABBIT.

Perhaps the famous children's story *The Velveteen Rabbit* can help us out. The story was written in 1922 by Margery Williams and describes the quest of a stuffed (fake) rabbit who becomes real through the love of its owner. There is much wisdom to be gleaned from this cute little story about the concept of realness. The rabbit felt it could truly become real when its owner loved it.

Perhaps men can truly become real when they love themselves and allow others to love them, instead of being in love with the image of themselves which seems to content society, media and themselves. When men question and reject the stereotypes, the cultural conditioning, the media and cultural hype, then they are free to create space to be themselves.

In the story, the rabbit becomes real when it sheds a tear. Perhaps men can become real when their inside feelings become congruent with their external expressions, when they shed tears and get beyond the emotional rigidity and polished presentation. The signs of realness may include moistness, softness, tenderness, sensuality, warmth and vulnerability. When these things are experienced perhaps the transformation from fake to real may begin.

BEING A 'REAL MAN' IS OFFICIALLY BAD FOR A MAN'S HEALTH

Catherine Bennett wrote an article in the Observer entitled 'It's time we ditched this bogus notion of real manhood'. In this article, Bennett refers to the results in a published report from the Samaritans entitled 'Men, Suicide and Society' which suggests society's expectations of men leads to high levels of depression, lack of self-worth and suicide.

The report highlights why the issue of 'real manhood' is a society issue and why a discourse on masculinity is essential. The report puts forward:

1. Men compare themselves against a 'gold standard', which prizes power, control and invincibility.
2. Men in mid-life are now part of the 'buffer' generation, not sure whether to be like their older, more traditional, strong, silent austere fathers or like their younger, more progressive, individualistic sons.
3. With the decline of traditional male industries, these men have lost not only their jobs but also a source of masculine pride and identity.
4. Men in midlife remain overwhelming dependant on a female partner for emotional support.

Bennett in her short article makes some pertinent points about the state of masculinity in UK society and the hierarchy of hegemonic masculinity. Hegemonic masculinity is described and characterized in the report as striving for power and dominance, aggression, courage, independency, efficiency, rationality, competitiveness, success, activity, control and invulnerability. This attitude will not perceive or admit anxiety, problems and burdens and withstands danger, difficulties and threats.

Bennett highlights how this 'gold standard' of hegemonic masculinity is being expressed by many men in society. She points to the example of 68-year old Sir Ranulph Fiennes, who at the time of the article was preparing another expedition to cross the Antarctic in winter. This 'old' man still sought to prove his 'Real' man status and his devotion to the traditional male ideal, honouring his 'balls of steel' knighthood, rather than the mere domesticity of being a father to his six-year-old daughter.

THE MESSAGES THAT WOMEN REGULARLY HEAR ABOUT BEING A WOMAN!

Women feel they have to prove their feminine status by fulfilling certain societal expectations. Women don't tend to be attacked on their gender or status of being a woman. But they will be judged on their appearance. They feel a need to fulfil the acceptable youthful beauty standards. Women are also judged on their body size. Many have been conditioned to behave in certain ways in order to be acceptable.

Women are under pressure to uphold strong social expectations of being the great and perfect mother who is maternal, caring, and nurturing at all times. Many mothers I have encountered through my work feel judged by not being good enough. They feel a societal pressure to be 'perfect'. They often feel guilty about their 'lack of'. Mothers feel like their children's actions and presentation could reflect badly on their mothering abilities and so may transmit high expectations onto their children.

There is still an expectation in society that women should be married (or at least in a stable relationship) and not have affairs. Their attitude should be pleasant, happy and amenable. They should be able to emote the full range of emotions with the exception of anger. Most women have had to endure a man telling her to 'Smile, it may never happen', so they learn to be a 'happy little girl for daddy'. If they stray from these expectations by acting assertively, not taking career breaks, having several sexual relationships, or not fulfilling the beauty standards, they could be met with a range of insults, including slut, whore, bossy, stubborn, bitch, ugly, aggressive cow, witch etc.

The message women often hear is that they should remain in their societal role and not move into the man's world. For some men, a strong, independent-minded woman can be a threat and can be emasculating.

EMOTIONAL FITNESS TOOLBOX

1. Reject the 'Real man' discourse by not using the phrases with other men or sons.

2. Take the Real Man test below. Women can take it in on behalf of your male partner, friend, brother, and father.

3. Awareness exercise: Observe men's behaviour around women, men and boys.

4. Question the status quo and the messages you hear from the media, peers and friends. When you hear people using these phrases — question them.

5. Talk to your friends. Tell them about the socially constructed messages you have heard, ask for their views.

THE REAL MAN TEST

Below are 30 indicators that will reveal your REAL man status — how REAL are you?

1. Siring many children — sowing your seed. The equation is more children = more man
2. Be hard — build a big strong body, be tough, rigid and impenetrable
3. Sexual conquests — be a stud, a sex god and live by this mantra — 'Find them, feel them, fuck them, forget them'
4. Be popular — make loads of mates never be a 'Billy no mates'
5. Be tough, angry and aggressive
6. Be cool, detached and distant (strong silent type)
7. Be successful financially — be a winner, be competitive — no losers allowed
8. Be powerful — achieve a high status/position in society or business
9. Ability to fight and look after yourself physically (evoke fear in others)
10. Remain in control — show no feelings (except anger) — Be stoical
11. Be big, be loud, be heard, be seen — demand attention

12. Be sacrificial — do heroic actions, be a hero
13. Be in possession of a big penis - size matters
14. Drink beer — lots of it
15. Big balls - Be a risk-taker — 'I dare you' — never back down
16. Eat beef — lots of it
17. Keep your body toned — achieve a six-pack/body image is important
18. Ability to banter, argue and have a superior intellect and rationality.
19. Love sport, play it, be good at it, watch it and be a winner
20. Be funny — make others laugh even if at others expense
21. Have the ability to protect others and fix their problems
22. Speed lover — drive fast & furious. Own a fast/ modified/big/expensive car.
23. Be attractive — have a beautiful woman (trophy) on your arm
24. Be in control (top-dog) in all situations
25. Ability to protect family and the honour of your mother
26. Ability to be practical, good at DIY

27. Work hard, work long, work smart & play hard
28. Own all the latest, expensive gadgets
29. Don't get too close to other men (unless when playing contact sport)
30. Be passive and unengaged when at home or with family

HOW DID HE DO?

Below 5: A complete fake
6 – 10: Unreal — grow some balls
11 – 20: Getting real but watch your back
21 – 30: You are the REAL thing, man!

ACTION

Once you've taken the test, reflect back on the five keys above. Do you feel any different now about the phrase, 'real man'? Are there any of the 30 points above you could work on in future?

KEY #3

SHAME IS THE SILENT TERROR

'Be Weak. Be Emotional. Be Vulnerable. Be Broken. Be whatever you feel with no shame at all. Know what you feel. You can't change what you are without knowing what you are.'

— MATT HAIG[26]

Toxic shame is a devious emotion. It likes to stay hidden but it lurks inside all men and is at the root of many emotional problems. It can be destructive because it inhibits men from growing. It imprisons them. It generates secretive aspects to male behaviour, leading them to isolated places where they can feel safe to expose their true selves. When toxic shame remains unseen it can be a main contributor to the trauma of emotional restriction. When left unaddressed, it is unlikely that growth will be long-lasting.

Toxic shame is embedded in the construction of masculinity. It is the weapon which keeps the hierarchy of patriarchy in power. Shame thrives when it is not exposed. Many of my clients have never considered how shame may be affecting their growth. When I mention the 'shame' word, my clients often become defensive and unsettled. They clearly feel uncomfortable with the word and its connotations.

Men are very often struggling with aspects of shame but it sends emotional shock waves through their sense of being. When they can begin to entertain it and in some ways accept it, they can find themselves riddled with it. It is like a cancer. Shame is often a key underlying issue and it is so important for men and women to face it. When clients are unable to work with shame, it may hinder the development of emotional fitness.

SHAME — A DEFINITION

The Cambridge online dictionary interprets shame in the three following ways:

> 1. *Personal inner shame at doing something wrong* — 'an uncomfortable feeling of guilt or of being ashamed because of your own, or someone else's bad behaviour'.
>
> 2. *A sense of shamelessness* — He said he felt no shame for what he had done.
>
> 3. *Externalized shame felt from others/society* — 'The children hung/bowed their heads in shame'. 'The shame of the scandal was so great that he shot himself a few weeks later' | 'You can't go out dressed like that — have you no shame'.

IS SHAME HEALTHY?

There is a difference between shame and toxic shame. The core of natural shame is to provide a 'consciousness', almost like having an internal eye which monitors behaviour and alerts the person to unhealthy choices. In her book, 'The Language of emotions', Karla McClaren says:

> **'Shame is a form of anger that arises when your boundary has been broken from the inside.'[27]**

A shame-filled person may express this internal anger through blushing and sweating. Shame assists in creating a well-regulated person by monitoring physical, emotional and spiritual desires. It's an internal guide that impacts on our emotions and our physical reactions. McClaren goes on to say:

> *'If you don't have conscious access to your free-flowing guilt and shame, you won't understand yourself, you'll be haunted by improper behaviours, addictions, and compulsions, and you'll be unable to stand upright at the centre of your psyche.'*[28]

Shame is your internal coach, bodyguard, and supervisor. If you can 'tune in' to its wisdom and internal nudges and remain in touch with its flow, it will effectively build character, maintain a healthy ego structure and help the individual to remain grounded. Healthy shame ultimately generates humility in which the person is in touch with who they are and know their strengths and weaknesses.

McLaren would suggest that to be shameless means to be out of touch with senses. This can lead to feeling out of control, out of touch and self-absorbed, resulting in limiting relational skills. People without shame are typically those who are unable to learn from their mistakes and stay on a loop of doing the same thing repeatedly hoping for a different outcome. They are essentially stuck on the shame cycle, but they can't see clearly what is happening and can't identify it. Alternatively, some people who refuse to live their lives according to cultural conditioning may appear shameless, uncaring or arrogant when in actual fact they are living according to their healthy internal shame antenna.

Many people find it extremely difficult to learn the lessons of authentic shame due to having to protect themselves from being shamed by others. Parents, teachers and authority figures can shame others when they feel out of control. McClaren explains that when a person is shamed externally, they can lose the ability to learn to moderate their own behaviours. She says,

> *'When we don't have a healthy connection to our own shame, we're often coerced into embodying other people's ideas of right and wrong'*[29]

GENDER ASSOCIATED SHAME

As discussed in the previous chapter, the 'Real man' discourse uses the weapon of shame to control men's expression of masculinity. Shame is used to attack men's gender by constantly questioning the status of their masculinity. The implication is they are not big enough, tough enough, man enough. The fear of being exposed, caught out or humiliated in any way makes men vigilant and 'on guard'. The best friend you can have is someone who 'has your back', a mate you can trust who will prevent someone emotionally 'knifing' you and will deflect attacks.

Toxic shame is often about being seen to be small or feeling small. Men strive to prevent 'smallness' in every way. Shame equals weakness, not fully reaching the standard

'It's a crying shame' is another phrase that's often used in society. Do not cry; it is shameful, weak and soft. I regularly hear boys shaming other boys by using terms such as 'pussy', 'gay' and 'girl'. These terms are used to attack another when there is any sign of difference, vulnerability or perceived weakness. These terms denigrate expressions of masculinity to a subordinate position.

I worked with a fourteen-year-old boy called Gary. He described himself as a 'street boy'. He fought his way through the world. His dad had left the family home after being violent to his mother. His brother was sadistically brutal to him, regularly beating him up and setting Gary up to take the consequences for his behaviour. This experience left him hardened, with anger clearly etched on his face.

During one session, Gary explicitly told me that he could never be perceived as weak or soft and could show no signs of weakness. His life motto, which he was able to clearly articulate to me, was 'kindness is weakness'. Gary struggled to trust anyone and often hurt others to try and get his needs met. I actually felt quite scared of him mixed with sadness and yet could understand why he would have this hardened view on life.

Kindness is weakness

Gary was angry and controlling. Unfortunately, without long-term support, I could see that he would hurt others. While working with him, he was able to share some of his pain and begin to trust me. He wrote poems and a rap full of his pain, wisdom and hope. Gary's honesty and trust in me made him vulnerable. During one session, he became tearful and not long after leaving my session, I heard he had got into trouble in the school by threatening another student. An older boy had looked at him in a way he found offensive and Gary ended up pushing a staff member out of the way to try and hit this other lad.

In her book 'I thought it was just me, but it isn't', Brene Brown explores shame and vulnerability. Her research is related to women and very insightful. However, she also discusses her work relating to men after she was questioned at a conference by a man, who said:

> *'We have shame, deep shame, but when we reach out and share our stories, we get the emotional shit beaten out of us... this is not just from other guys but from women as well... you say you want us to be vulnerable and real... but in reality you can't stand it. It makes you sick to see us like that.'*[30]

This is a common story. I have heard similar comments many times from men. Even though many women want men to be emotionally available, they still want their man to be strong and protective. I suspect this has something to do with the deep societal and psychological connection to the prince/princess patriarchal story mentioned earlier on in this book.

After the encounter with the man at the conference, Brene Brown was inspired to do some research about the way men are shamed. She spent some time working with a group of young men who felt they had to deal with shame by 'looking like they can kick someone's ass.' In her research, Brown discovered that messages and expectations around masculinity are often driven by shame.

Men are shamed if they are perceived to show any kind of weakness or failure

Some of the definitions Brown recorded from the participants included:

> *Shame is failure. At work, on the football field, in your marriage, in bed, with money, with your children.*
>
> *Shame is being wrong. Not doing it wrong but being wrong.*
>
> *Shame happens when people think you are soft. It's degrading and shaming to be seen as anything but tough.*
>
> *Revealing any weakness is shaming. Basically, shame is weakness.*
>
> *Showing fear is shameful. You cannot show fear. You cannot be afraid.*
>
> *Our worst fear is being criticised or ridiculed – either one of these is extremely shaming.*[31]

When men feel shame or are told they should be ashamed, what they hear is: I'm weak, I'm a failure, I'm not a man. They hear this ringing deep within themselves and it is the core of the compass of male toxic shame (see below).

When we hurt, we hurt others!

Men and women will transmit their toxic shame; they will project it on to someone else and then feel shame for behaving in this sort of way.

THE COMPASS OF MALE TOXIC SHAME

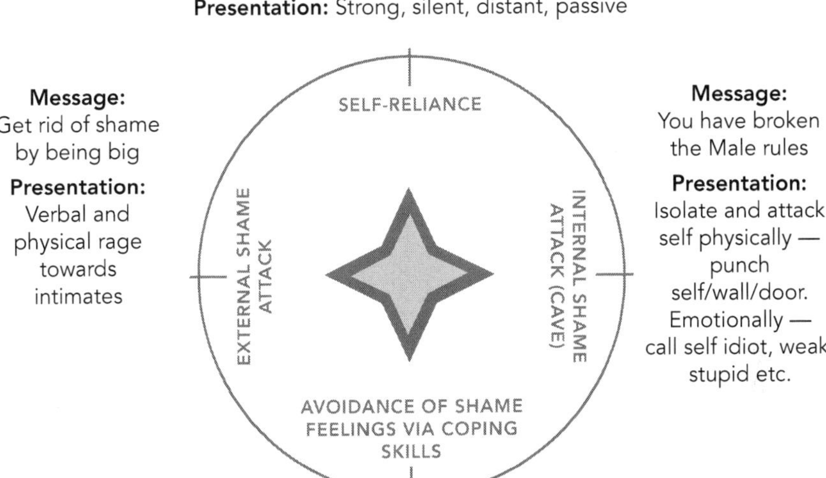

The power of this gender-associated shame leaves boys and men traumatised. Men are under huge pressure to appear tough, strong, stoic, powerful, successful, fearless, in control and knowledgeable. Shame reduces emotional expression by shutting down clear external communication. This hidden force takes the shame-based person back to old survival strategies which are often based in anger.

THE TERROR OF THE MALE CODE (MAN RULES)

'Toxic shame' and the 'Male code' (otherwise known as the male rules), are cut from the same cloth as mechanisms of control. When men obey the code and maintain the status quo, it keeps them in the box. The box isolates a man, it breeds negative thoughts and convinces him that if he questions the code, he will be seen as weird, abnormal or unnatural. Likewise, toxic shame tells men there is only one way to be a man and if you deviate from this path you are at risk of being isolated, bullied and ostracized.

To remain inside the box, to feel like they are fitting in, and to prevent shame, men have had to develop a robust coping strategy, which usually means fostering the inner tyrant. The tyrant will give the man a good beating if he dares to step out of line. The inner tyrant fills men's heads (of course women know the same inner tyrant as well) with a constant stream of questioning, to criticise any action that could cause shame. The tyrant will seek to control the man by constantly using the commands of 'should', 'could', 'ought' and 'must'. The tyrant will terrorise the man into obedience, with the ultimate threat of being ostracised from the tribe.

Many men have become experts at mustabation!!

Dr. Michael Obsatz describes how this process leads to shame-based masculinity and how this impacts on boys and men.

> *"Millions of boys are shamed into fitting into a model of masculinity. They are called sissy, wimp, wuss, momma's boy (etc), if they do not conform to a cultural norm. In the process of conforming, boys lose a part of themselves, and spend their lives grieving these losses. Rather*

than being allowed to authentically develop into their true selves, they are coerced into a narrow 'blueprint' of masculinity."[32]

Herb Goldberg, in his book *The New Male*, written in 1979, says this "blueprint for masculinity is a blueprint for self-destruction." This shaming process means that boys experience loss if they do fit in. It is a no-win proposition.[33]

Obsatz[34] lists the messages boys and men receive:

THERE ARE AT LEAST TWENTY-FIVE MESSAGES BOYS ARE TAUGHT

1. Sexualize affection — all touch is sexual touch
2. Have many sexual conquests
3. Maintain a strong image
4. Prove manhood by taking risks, even if foolish
5. Don't be a virgin
6. Don't be vulnerable
7. Don't cry
8. Don't express fear
9. Don't ask for help, guidance or directions
10. Don't trust anyone
11. Be disposable - be willing to die for your country
12. Pretend to know even when you don't
13. Act tough
14. Be in control
15. Dominate others
16. Devalue what is "feminine" in yourself and others
17. Be emotionally detached
18. Tough it out

19. Don't take care of your body
20. Win at all costs
21. Abuse your body
22. More is better - money, sex, food, alcohol
23. Objectify women
24. Prove manhood
25. You are what you achieve or accomplish

THE GENDER SECURITY SERVICE

Gender security for many men is very fragile. It causes men to be on their guard and hyper-vigilant. Men have to be watchful so they are not caught acting in any way unlawfully with the 'Real Men' police ready to issue any gender-bending with a gender shaming ticket. Men must be ready to ward off any attack that could associate them with the 'other' gender. The 'gender police' will shame a perpetrator by accusing them of being a woman or associating them with women's genitalia.

Boys and men will be attacked if they are or appear too close to their Mum, with the constant attack of 'Mummy's Boy' an accusation that the boy might need Mummy to protect him. On the other hand, the playground banter attack on another boy is often 'your mum' which includes an attack on her as a sexual object and could include insulting her looks or accusing the boy of being a 'motherfucker' or threatening him on how they will have sex with her.

At this stage, the gender police, in the form of peers, is training boys that emotional intimacy with women is not acceptable and that women are now sexual objects. To have intimacy with women now means sex. But remaining emotionally intimate with their mother risks keeping the boy soft or turning him into a woman.

As you can see, this is a very confusing time for boys. They are caught in the middle of different perspectives, wanting to be independent, uncertain about their own needs, conscious of how they appear yet wanting the support of their parents. The boy wants to protect his mother, protect himself and deep down wants to preserve an intimate connection. Boys are caught in the tension of letting go of the connection with the 'feminine' which can result in unhealthy expressions of pushing Mum away. This could typically include verbally abusing her, pushing her affection and warmth away and seeking to prove that he does not need her.

Inside his home, the boy is seeking to separate from the mother, and outside the home, he is learning that he has to protect her

---

This interplay generates an incredible amount of information which feeds into gender conditioning and division. The crucial (and traumatic) messages many boys learn at this stage is that emotional intimacy is soft and this is what women do. Secondly, vulnerable emotions must remain hidden. Thirdly, they learn that 'sex equals intimacy' — the main way to connect and get close to women is via sex and hence women become sexual objects.

What does it mean to be a man? Not to be a woman!

Obsatz[35] describes how gender shaming can affect a boy's development. He lists the losses boys endure generating developmental trauma:

1. Loss of intimate connection to mother and father
2. Loss of emotional outlets — crying, showing fear
3. Loss of trust in other males who betray, tease or shun them
4. Loss of the option to be gentle, nurturing, vulnerable
5. Loss of the freedom to make mistakes
6. Loss of internal awareness and emotional disconnection
7. Loss of power over one's own destiny
8. Loss of freedom to give and receive non-sexual affection

THE UNHEALTHY SHAME SURVIVAL TOOLKIT

Having explored how men experience shame, we now need to consider how men manage and cope with shame. Below, I have highlighted men's six unhealthy shame survival strategies.

1. Defend

When men feel threatened, their emotional defence system can be triggered, automatically closing their internal psychological shutters. Many men quickly become defensive. This classic default state men adopt is about keeping their distance and appearing almost robotic with their responses. It is possible sometimes to literally see some men's eyes glaze over. The shutters descend. They withdraw. In this position, men will revert to the safety of the cognitive and rational, with a typical response being 'Stick to the facts'. Feelings will be relegated as unimportant and untrustworthy. They feel the need to be right.

2. Denial & disguise

Another way for men to keep shame at bay is through denial. 'It's not my fault' is the common refrain. Men have learnt to protect themselves by refusing to take responsibility for their actions. This can result in men struggling to utter words like 'sorry', 'I made a mistake' and 'I don't know'. Admitting this kind of vulnerability would be an admission that he is 'less than' a real man and he could risk being flooded with shame, which is too much to bear. Men who use this tool may appear emotionally fragile and disguise it through substance misuse. Some men who use this strategy may become addicted. They may be told that they have addictive personalities.

3. Destroy and distort

Boys and men learn that the best form of defence is offence. Meet attack with attack. When you feel shame, shame back — and so the cycle continues. Banter is, of course, a culturally accepted and conditioned way of continuing the shame cycle. It can often be the only form of communication men have! If the threat to his fragile emotional equilibrium becomes too much, it has to be attacked. Once the attack is dealt with he can return to his survival state. Men who use this tool may behave aggressively and may need to maintain a sense of control.

4. Disappear

Toxic shame can lead to a man feeling 'less than' and small. His strategy here is to vanish. This is difficult because he feels a conflict between NOT being noticed and wanting to BE noticed. This position is rooted in the fear of being humiliated and embarrassed. Men and boys in this position protect themselves by tucking an emergency cloak of invisibility in their back pocket to use in possible shaming situations. When events produce risk, men who use this tactic will adopt a passive approach, fade into the background, go quiet, freeze and will literally hope they can't be seen and so disappear.

This shame survival tool can moor men on the margins of situations and life, leaving them observing the action and ultimately feeling stuck and possibly chronically bored. When boys and men utter the words 'everything is boring' this can be translated as 'everything is risky if he dares to move from his frozen position'. This passive shame, protective approach can lead to men, externally and internally, isolating themselves, leading to mental health and relational issues.

This strategy taps into his deep self-reliance and the cave/shed mentality is the obvious outcome. The physical and psychological 'shed' is seen as a safe place but can actually just perpetuate the shame cycle. When a man feels he has been shamed or he has 'lost' it by shaming others, he may retreat to the cave where he psychologically licks his wounds, picks off old scabs and gives himself an internal beating. He applies a form of band-aid before leaving the shed and re-entering the situation where the shame incident occurred. This incident is often 'moved on from', 'forgotten' and not referred to again. He carries on stuffing down shame incidents and the cycle of shame begins the loop once again.

5. Dissociation

This is closely connected to the 'disappear' strategy. This primitive survival tool is often practised subconsciously, where one typically separates body and mind. In many ways, we all do this every day. For example, when we drive a car our bodies work automatically and our minds can be on something else. At that point, our internal and external worlds are incongruent. A person may be physically present but internally he could be elsewhere. The man utilising this tool would typically be found 'zoning out', appear distant and emotionally unengaged. The man may come across as silent, passive and unengaging.

6. Daring and determination

'I dare you' is a common game boys play which is often about proving their right to be part of the male club. 'He who dares wins' is the SAS motto. It describes how men perceive 'daring' to be the road to success and the route to being part of an elite force. The SAS are the most feared fighting force in the world. This 'more than' survival skill is a great disguise for shame.

The successful one bolsters the defence against shame attacks. This can also be true for men in business — they strive to achieve and become important, powerful and noticed as a way of deflecting any sense of smallness and shame. Many men using this tool may become 'addicted' to their work, striving to maintain the status they have gained. This strategy can also lead to ruin. A man may stretch values and morals through sexual encounters, gambling and risky business practices.

SHAME IS TERRORISING MEN

If men are to grow in maturity, they must encounter the damage that has been done through the trauma of shame. Krugman discusses three causes in the development of shame, with particular reference to male development.

1. Shame is generated in the boy when he becomes aware that his parents react negatively to parts of himself.
2. The second encounter with shame is when the boy/teenager/man is unable to live up to the male code and stereotypes.

3. Thirdly, shame emerges through family dysfunction, particularly if it includes domestic violence and alcoholism.[36]

IS DEPRESSION A COVER FOR SHAME?

Most statistics tell us that women are more depressed than men. What the statistics fail to tell us is that the data depends on patients going to the doctor to receive help and men tend to attend medical centres less often. This means the statistics are skewed. This sense of dis-ease and failure to function can often be squeezed out through the big, tough, strong emotion of anger or sucked inwards, generating depressive tendencies. Shame is a powerful emotion and if it isn't brought into awareness and expressed it can stick around in the psyche and body.

Obsatz believes that, deep down, men find it very hard to manage intense shame. The loss of male emotional expression means that men will generally 'act out' as a way of disguising this loss in some way. Men will, however, often find themselves stuck on the cycle of rage and shame, externalising their inner pain through the following ways:

1. Violence against men, women and children
2. Deaths due to foolish risk-taking
3. Addictions to numb out pain
4. Depression, isolation and loneliness
5. Injuries and deaths due to men's sports — racing, boxing, etc.

IS SHAME THE SILENT AND SECRET KILLER OF MEN?

Up to thirteen men take their own lives in the UK every day. Thirteen men get to such a bad place, internally, that they feel life is no longer worth living. Some men will come to therapy and begin the steps needed for change. Remember, you are taking steps just by reading this book or giving it on to someone.

Suicide is the biggest killer of men between the ages of 20-49. More men kill themselves than die by car accidents, cancer and heart disease

---

The financially poorest of men are ten times more likely to kill themselves than those from richer backgrounds. The tragedy is that few people are aware of this. Political intervention is often non-existent.

If we were to put this into perspective, here is the cold, hard truth. We live in a society which pours huge amounts of money into combatting the external terrorist threat. Meanwhile, the internal terror men face is killing them in vast numbers. To put these numbers in context:

- During the years of the Afghanistan war, 458 UK soldiers were killed in battle and 179 men lost their lives in the Iraq war.
- Throughout 2011-12, there were 564 murders in the UK.
- In 2016 in the UK, nearly 5000 men died by their own hands.

The suicide figure is huge, but the media coverage of it is minimal. If 5000 men were being killed or murdered every year or were killed at war, then it would be on the national agenda. Why aren't the suicide numbers getting the publicity they deserve?

Shame and suicide are closely linked. Why isn't suicide talked about in society? Perhaps the answer is that it generates societal shame. We don't want to admit this is happening. We don't want to ask the uncomfortable questions and perhaps admit the unpalatable truths that might emerge. Perhaps it just feels too shameful to mention and this is a national disgrace. Instead, societies and politicians avoid it and do very little to address the causes. Ultimately as a nation, the shame survival toolkit outlined above is employed on a national level.

SHAME AND HIGH-RISK BEHAVIOURS

I recall a client telling me that a friend hung himself in his family home. Apparently, he had been struggling with some difficult emotions but was unable to find the help that he needed. Friends did not know the extent of his inner turmoil, nobody could understand how he got to the point of taking his own life. His death left his family in distress and friends wondered how they could have done more to help.

One of my young clients, a fifteen-year-old boy was talking to me about how he tried to take his own life. He had been struggling with feeling down, lacking energy and feeling insecure about his friendships. At the time of his suicide attempt, he felt very isolated and had been constantly regurgitating negative feelings. He was stuck on the loop of the shame cycle.

It is increasingly becoming evident that many men carry some dark secrets. One such terrible secret is the trauma of sexual abuse or rape hidden inside for so long they can no longer bear the shame of it all. They can see no other way of being relieved of this awful inner pain and the shame leads to self-destruction.

Krugman suggests that unbearable shame feelings are associated with high-risk behaviours especially suicide, which may have some bearing on the mystery of 'normal' men committing violence to self and others.

The man code and the messages men hear about masculinity are slowly killing men. Shame does not respect external strength and festers in silence and isolation. As mentioned elsewhere, self-reliance creates a perfect place for shame to thrive. Increasingly my work with men is about working with shame. A core practice of this work is de-shaming. This means to normalise a man's internal world and to let him know he is not the only one who struggles with feelings of shame.

When men live internally isolated lives, shame has free reign; it's like a cancer, growing inside them and it is very destructive. When men talk to other men and are authentic, it is almost like one can hear an existential sigh escaping from their soul. They breathe out and start to release their shame. This is a great moment, a big step towards authenticity. To counter the shaming culture, we need both men and women to take responsibility for their gender-associated expectations and stereotypes and model non-shameful communication. We need to understand how our expectations of gender forces a straitjacket onto emotional expression.

THE HEALTHY SHAME RESILIENT TOOLKIT

Developing shame resilience is not easy. It will take disciplined emotional exercise. The good news is, however, that becoming shame-resilient is possible. The tools I will describe below have worked on my own shame-based behaviour and have been effective in helping many of my clients.

1. Work on welcoming authentic shame into your life

People with a lack of authentic shame are unable to take responsibility for their actions; they seem to expect other people to accept them no matter what. They are often reluctant to reflect on their actions and to apologise when they get things wrong. I have seen this played out so often, especially within the relational work that I do.

Jack and Charlotte were in their first session with me. Charlotte was absolutely fed up with Jack for not taking responsibility for his behaviour regarding a lack of input to family and home matters. Jack expressed his anger at Charlotte's request, complaining he was so busy at work and how could she expect him to do anymore. He was unable to welcome authentic shame into his life at this point.

By verbalising her complaint, Charlotte was looking after her boundaries by not being prepared to allow Jack to disrespect her. Jack was displaying leaky internal boundaries, wanting acceptance from his partner without taking responsibility for his actions. If Charlotte refused to challenge Jack, her trust in her internal senses would be weakened allowing the other to dictate. In building shame resilience, it is essential to maintain strong boundaries around people who express unhealthy shame.

Quit spending time worrying about what others think of you. How you think and feel about them is what matters

---

McLaren offers friends three chances to take responsibility for their behaviour. If the friend offends and does not take responsibility for her behaviour and continues to behave without shame, she will give them a strike. After three strikes, she will prepare herself to walk away from that relationship. Strong internal and external boundaries are essential to maintain connection to senses and protection against others' shame loop.

'Authentic shame is essential to your health and your relationships — you won't feel happy without it.'[37]

---

2. Become a shame buster

Discovering toxic shame and raising awareness of it, is really important in your work to become shame resilient. Shame keeps itself well-hidden and is very subtle. It thrives in darkness. You may not even have recognised it, as it may have been part of your inner fabric for so long. Wake up to the sound and feel of shame in your words and in your body, identify it and shine a torch on it, bring it into the light. Start to notice the triggers of your shame. What are the words, gestures and people who provoke a sense of smallness or humiliation? Once you start to do this, you will become more aware of shame and how it works.

Not until we identify and accept the presence of shame can we start to tackle its corrosive presence in our lives. One of the deeper ways shame can manipulate us is through self-sabotage. I discovered this regular internal script later on in life. When the toxic voice inside me whispered, 'I shouldn't exist', my internal thinking was that I had no right to be successful and affirmed.

When I subconsciously found myself with the possibility of being successful, I would discreetly sabotage the opportunity. Typically, this would mean I would make an excuse or avoid an important meeting. I would not push myself forward, inhibit myself and hide. I would then go back on the shame cycle of berating myself. The acceptance of shame in itself can be a big breakthrough.

3. Name it and shame it

Do you find yourself saying negative things to yourself internally? Do you call yourself an idiot, stupid, useless, fool, pointless or feel that 'your opinion doesn't matter' and 'you're a mistake'? When we know the names and words of shame and capture those words then they cease to have so much power over us. Work on the following tips:

- Say your shame words aloud to yourself, get to know them and listen to how they feel.
- Stop beating yourself up. 'Capture' those negative words and stop 'calling' or bullying yourself; refuse to say negative words to

yourself. Stop agreeing with the shame words. Question them and challenge them.

- Let yourself off the hook. Seek to replace the shaming words with positive words and phrases such as 'it's okay', 'I made a mistake', 'I'm not the only one', 'just try again', this takes emotional discipline and perseverance, but will build resilience to shame.
- Develop self-compassion. Practise affirming yourself and developing a positive inner discourse or self-talk. Learn to trust your feelings and stay in touch with your authentic shame. Develop self-empathy and be kind to yourself.

4. Practise de-shaming in public

Take a risk and self-disclose. Those who self-disclose are more likely to have friends who self-disclose. When you talk to others about your feelings and share vulnerabilities, it can be contagious. This is why therapeutic group work is so useful where we can finally realise that I'm not the only one who struggles with shame. In fact, it is very common.

5. Ask for feedback from your friends

Directly ask for feedback. 'What do you think of me?' This is another risky exercise but important for growth. If your friends cannot manage this kind of relationship — get some different friends.

6. People watch

Observe other people's shame and pick up shame cues when people are integrating with others and practise empathy. When you notice adults shaming children or other adults — have a word with them.

7. Become aware of your anger and rage triggers

Listen to your body and feelings, such as blushing and a sense of feeling small.

8. Public shame

Defend yourself. When people shame you in public try practicing assertiveness and let them know what they are doing is not acceptable. Try not to absorb the external shame — renounce it. Work out some ready-made stock statements you can use in any given context such as, 'I don't like the way you are talking to me!' or 'I feel hurt when you treat me like that.'

9. Book an appointment with a therapist

In therapy, you will begin to get in touch with your inner thoughts and shame. Increasingly much of my work with clients is around shame. However, in my work with men, many of them will refuse to go anywhere near shame. They almost physically shudder when it is mentioned. I would also encourage male clients to work with a male therapist. This can be challenging for men due to the risk of shame exposure. A good therapist will offer empathy, warmth and a non-judgemental attitude.

10. Men, join a men's group. Women, join a women's group

Group work increases learning fast and is one of the best ways of de-shaming and addressing toxic shame.

EMOTIONAL FITNESS TOOLBOX

1. De-shame — Practise reminding yourself that your inner story is the story of the majority of women/men. 'I thought it was only me but it isn't.'

2. Practise some shame-busting, identify and capture those shame words/feelings.

3. Develop self-compassion and letting yourself off the hook.

4. Work on the rest of the shame resilient toolkit.

5. Read Brene Brown's book — 'I thought it was only me, but it isn't!' This is about how we experience difficult feelings around shame. The book shows us that everybody else is struggling with similar feelings.

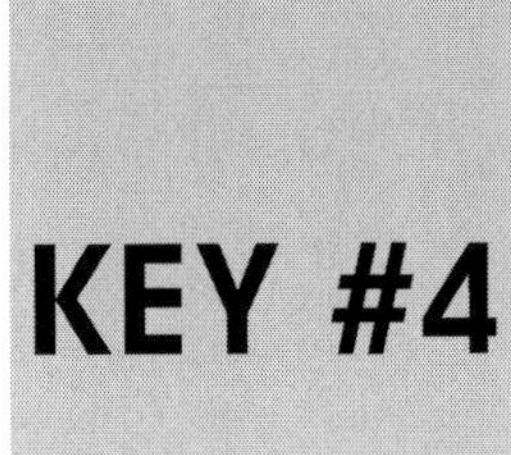

KEY #4

SIZE REALLY DOES MATTER

'Small boys create the biggest problems'

The 'small man syndrome' may not be a scientifically proven concept but it appears it may have some truth in it. Little men often feel they need to prove themselves.

Whilst it is often said, 'it's not the size that matters, it is what you do with it that counts' or 'it's quality not quantity' that matters, these pithy little sayings count for nothing when related to men's feelings regarding their physical size and the size of their penis. How men actually feel about their size can have a big impact on their self-esteem and confidence.

IT IS NOT JUST ABOUT PENIS SIZE

It is not just about penis size but in the world of the 'real man' discourse, it is difficult for many men to ignore. For millennia, men have been concerned and sensitive about the size of their penis and how this reflects on their manhood. In Neolithic art, men's virility and penis size were grossly exaggerated, monstrous and almost god-like. It appeared that men sensed that they should be led by their penis.

Penis size is never far from men's internal thought processes and features regularly in men's magazines and internet discussions. Sometimes, penis size is in the news. A few years ago, a story appeared on the BBC website in reference to the size of condoms. It remained one of the 'most viewed' articles for some time. It was announced that some nations need bigger and smaller condom sizes to make safer sex more possible.

Okay, that's the penis out of the way. Well, not quite. I'm sure we will come back to this important male member. But essentially this chapter is about how 'smallness' in any context for men is usually perceived as a negative and possibly a shaming thing. For many men to feel safe in their manhood, they need to feel big in any way they can. This will help them to feel more secure in their masculinity.

BIG MAN

Many men like everything in their life to be big and are driven to make it bigger. This may include a big body, a big bank account, a big house or a big family. They may want to command a big job, with a high and powerful position. Some men may want a big intellect with a large number of knowledge feeding a big ego.

Men may want a big car, demand big respect and are only feel satisfied with a woman with big breasts. In this 'big' world, they demand to be seen and noticed. If they are unable to be a big shot or successful in business then they will seek to be big in gangs, have a large amount of sexual conquests, be a top fighter (the big man), or create a rigid and huge body.

To be BIG is powerful and will earn the recipient BIG respect?

Even as I write this book, there is a part of me doing it because I want my thoughts, experience and knowledge to go out into the world. I want to be noticed and applauded. I want to be seen as successful. I want ultimately, to be bigger than I am or feel I am now. The need to externalise, to go into the world is strong. In many ways this is a natural human desire, yet when it feeds something deeper then it may not be so healthy.

A delegate who attended one of my workshops mentioned he had read research about the way babies were held by adults. The research stated that babies were often held according to gender. Male babies were positioned in baby slings looking away from the holder's body, while female babies were held with their faces towards the parent's body. Perhaps even at this tender age, boys and girls pick up messages regarding internalising and externalising.

Men's need to do things 'bigger and better' goes beyond the personal and into society and space. Many men appear to have an insatiable appetite for greatness: from conquering the highest mountain or creating the tallest phallic-shaped skyscraper to acquiring larger amounts of territory.

Throughout thousands of years, men seem to have a need to dominate. It's almost always men who are dictators. Men are on an insatiable quest to explore space and the final frontier. Clearly this drive is not just a negative energy, through this longing for new, more and bigger, men have been at the root of many amazing innovations and new technologies which have made life far easier, happier and more palatable.

HOW HAS BIG BECOME SO IMPORTANT TO MEN?

I am left with several questions about the male desire for big, bigger, biggest. Is their thirst for greatness part of a man's DNA? Is it in their genes and at the core of man's essential being? Is this internal drive connected to social conditioning and the lack of psychological 'bigness' they feel inside? Where does this appetite for greatness spring from?

Is it purely biological and linked to the penis, is it actually 'in their jeans?'

Perhaps it won't be long before a gene is found which backs up the view that men can't stop wanting to be big or having a desire for power over others. Perhaps it is pure instinct, which is how some men view their sexual pursuits saying, 'it wasn't my fault', ' it's instinct', 'it's the way I was made', 'I can't do anything about this force within me',' it has a life of its own.' I think the way our bodies are formed does have a psychological impact on our way of being. Within a holistic approach to life, physiology and psychology cannot be separated.

A man's genitalia is on the outside of his body. Psychologically, this may indicate that men are naturally more comfortable living life on the outside and therefore find it harder to discover what is going on inside of them. The penis also changes shape and size, from flaccid to erect, with the erect penis or phallus full of potency, rigidity, virility and power. Does the phallus generate a need for external power and 'lead' men to penetrate further into things, places and ways of being? Does the phallus generate men towards hardness, greater height, to build and rise up? Does it require to be seen, to be noticed and to leave a legacy?

Being BIG = safety

For many men, the feeling of generating an erection not only brings comfort and pleasure, it also has a sense of power and this can be addictive. Perhaps the phallic feeling of bigness, potency and power spills over into other areas of their lives. This great feeling eventually turns into a philosophy of life and a way of seeing and constructing the world. For a man who may feel small inside, this unsatisfactory feeling can generate a sense of weakness and inferiority.

This feeling may be translated into the opposite polarity of bigness and domination. Feeling small may feel unsafe and hence, to feel big will generate a sense of safety and control. Being at the top, having power over others and living within a hierarchical culture creates comfort. This can lead to a sense that authoritarianism is safe, fundamentalism is safe, institutionalism is safe, dualism is safe and patriarchy is safe. Being small is unsafe — physically, socially, intellectually and emotionally.

Being emotional = unsafe

Men generally 'feel' unsafe around the expression of a full range of emotions. Many men believe they are in control of their emotions, but they can often 'lose their temper' that big emotion they have relied on to protect them.

Patriarchy is a coping strategy for men who feel unsafe and small. It is a system based on insecurity and fear. It generates a hierarchy of power around gender, sexuality and culture. Patriarchy is a worldwide male coping skill, or a male-code sanctioned by those with the most power.

If you stick to the code, you will be safe. If you deviate from the code and question this sacred male pact by living differently, be it a different sexuality, not acting macho enough, being un-sporty or are unwilling to play the power game, then you will be punished and possibly ostracized from the male community.

Failing to build emotional muscle, will ultimately keep men internally small. The 'inner boy' will never grow up, leaving this child-like persona to dominate the adult male life

---

I have worked with numerous clients who exhibit this way of being. One such man, let us call him Tony, is very successful in his business life, but has struggled to maintain a healthy and successful relationship. He has found it hard to sleep well and for the past twenty years, he has felt stuck in a loop, repeating the same behaviour, replaying the same script.

Tony feared rejection and he managed this by wanting to maintain control in his relationships which resulted in the lack of depth or growth with partners. This has resulted in the same relational patterns emerging and when he came to see me, he was feeling hopeless. It emerged during our sessions that Tony had been internally hoarding his anger and he found himself stuck in the eternal boy with a sense of 'it's not fair' and 'poor me'.

After the third session, he began to entertain that when he was a boy he had many unmet emotional needs and he had created a coping strategy which appeared to work but in fact was restricting him. His internal boy was hurting and he sought to manage that hurt by achieving externally. But it wasn't the answer; for all his external achievement, he remained unfulfilled. In trying to get his needs met, Tony became stuck in the same consciousness that actually created his hurt and was metaphorically banging his head against a brick wall. The internal pain was so bad he was planning to withdraw from pursuing further relationships.

STAYING 'BIG' IS A SOURCE OF GREAT STRESS

The problem with striving to sustain the position that makes a man 'big' or powerful is that it is exhausting. It demands a huge amount of time and effort and a constant sense of remaining watchful. The risk is that someone will take your position. Striving for external 'bigness' is stressful because you are ultimately not the biggest.

Some men strive to be the biggest man on the block. He is left watching his back, concerned someone bigger will emerge

---

Keeping the top position is stressful. Men are often caught in the trap of needing to protect their external success and achievements. He can't afford to stand still, otherwise, he may become smaller. This is the root of the competitive or driven male. Life becomes competition; it is the only way to stay on top. Clinging to the top position is driven by fear and this is the same feeling that drove them to the top in the first place.

It is at this point that 'bigness' can become addictive. The need for more money, bigger and more houses, bigger land and profits and more growth can become compulsive. Before you know it, the drive takes over, many lose touch with reality and the need to fulfil the 'lack' of inside or the smallness inside gobbles up any external advantage. At this point, life can appear meaningless and soulless.

The market is driven by continual growth. Profit must continue at all costs. To fulfil the capitalist machine, more raw resources must be consumed to produce a constant stream of 'new' and 'big', with profit continuing at all costs. The consumer feeds on a need to have the latest gadget, leading to gadget/wealth/material obesity. This generates inequality between the haves and the have nots and ultimately between the inner and exterior world. This ultimately generates a disturbance in individuals and societies.

IS SMALL REALLY BEAUTIFUL?

To embrace our smallness is the biggest obstacle most men have to overcome. Few people are happy with external smallness. If the body doesn't grow at the perceived developmental rate, then the child may be given growth hormones or other interventions. Cosmetic surgery is now very common for women who want bigger breasts and for men in enlarging the penis, bigger muscles or muscle definition. All of the above is, of course, related to physical growth, where is the medication for the lack of psychological growth?

Small is not something western society gives much credence to, but small does appear to be beautiful in a few areas in modern society. Technological advances have generated keyhole surgery and the ability to make ever more powerful and increasingly smaller/slimmer communication gadgets. Small waist sizes (size zero!) are marketed as 'the ideal' for women. Cosmetic surgery is also used to make body parts smaller, including breasts, noses, stomachs and to create more defined abs. Otherwise, everything is about getting bigger!

I feel big by 'making' others feel small — the bullying epidemic

---

For some men, being 'big' unfortunately involves picking on men (or women) further down the pecking order. This could involve banter, patronising language and disrespect. This 'pecking order' game-playing could fluctuate all day long, with the same men assuming 'less than' and 'more than' positions.

When a man feels that he has been in the 'less than' position he may feel the need to be in a 'power-over' position in another relationship; in this way the bullied becomes the bully. He may end up projecting his hurt onto his partner, child, pet, or venting at the referee. He may self-punish or bully himself either physically or internally — putting himself down through destructive self-talk or through physical self-harming and getting stuck on the shame cycle. This hierarchy and pecking order may have been learnt in the family home.

'TOP DOG' MESSAGES LEARNT FROM THE FAMILY HOME

Whenever a parent, teacher or another adult calls a child 'stupid' they set up the top-dog system, alerting the child to the fact that there is a pecking order of esteem and according to them, the child has failed. When a father mocks and shames his son, the little boy learns power is the way to protect internal and external smallness. Whenever a parent or a big person patronises, belittles and disrespects a child, this pecking order game is reinforced. When children's opinions are not sought, whenever their voice is not heard or they are not included, this dualistic system will thrive.

Today, we are much more aware of bullying and the impact it can have on the individual. Many schools will support anti-bullying week, businesses have grievance procedures to empower and protect employees. However, as schools have become increasingly larger, with huge peer groups, bullying has become harder to control; it can creep in, sometimes in subtle ways. Low level bullying has become an acceptable part of life. It is commonplace for children, young people and adults to be 'put down', mocked, verbally abused and increasingly physically threatened.

The Golden Rule - 'treat others as you would like to be treated', appears to have lost its appeal and is not to be trusted. Many young people have already learnt that they will 'feel' bigger or better than others if they can 'make' others feel small. This feeling is, of course, short-lived. The sad thing about the top dog system is that deep down these young people live by the motto 'bully or be bullied'. Ultimately, there are no winners. No one is happy. Everyone just ends up surviving, doing what they can to get through.

THE TOP FOUR WAYS MEN JOIN THE CULT OF BIG

1. Body Building

Recent years have seen a surge in men and teenage boys concerned with having the right shaped body and the essential six-pack. I worked with a fourteen-year-old boy who was obsessed with body and was constantly taking selfies. He went to a gym several nights a week and was proud of his honed muscles and 'ripped' body. He had also developed a distaste for pubic hair! This lad was living proof of the 'spornosexual'.

The body has become a project and some men have become obsessive about the way they look. When I observe boys and men involved in bodybuilding, I am left asking two questions. Is bodybuilding and obsessive body sculpting covering up their inner emotional flabbiness? Is the body the best cover for inner smallness and fragility?

It is also important to note there is an increasing usage of drugs and steroids to enhance sports ability and bodybuilding. Men are harming themselves and becoming addicted in order to be big.

2. Being successful

In today's culture success normally means financial success. This is evident at an international and national level, in which most countries measure their success through their national GDP and economic growth. The goal of success consumes social media sites, including LinkedIn in which people will declare their success by standing next to a fast car, massive boat or an oversized house.

The cult of BIG is fed by the gods of speed, size and success

---

These successful people will then be keen to tell you how you can be like them. I responded to this vacuous nonsense by posting a message about my friend Duncan Dyason:

'One of the most successful people I know is not rich. He does not have a massive house, a flashy car or an enormous boat. Yet, he is an amazing entrepreneur. He is an author with friends all over the globe and received an MBE for his work. I am proud to call this man my friend. He is successful because he devotes himself to developing innovative and effective projects in helping street children in Guatemala. He has raised a huge amount of money and made thousands of people aware of this problem.'

3. Body enhancements

My spam box fills up with emails about how I could enhance my manhood by having a penis the size of a baseball bat and offering me procedures for other body enhancements. These emails seek to convince me that by being bigger, I will somehow be more attractive and successful with women. Big body parts are now possible even if you are not naturally endowed. Now you can recline on the operating table and wake up a new man.

4. Big Business

As previously mentioned in this chapter, achievement is everything. Get to the top, however you can. If it means stepping on others, cheating and lying, just do it, because the top is all that matters. When you are at the top you have power, position and privilege and can look down on all the 'little' people.

THE UNMET NEEDS OF THE INTERNAL BOY CAN DOMINATE THE ADULT MAN

External bigness in the way I have described often hides internal smallness. If the unmet needs of the internal boy are not met or heard then the inner boy ends up dominating the man. This leads to the formation of the 'adult boy'.

Deep inside the adult boy is fear. Men fear exposure. They are scared they will be found out, that people will see they are putting on an act

---

Men fear someone will discover their vulnerability — their flaws, mistakes, inabilities, insecurities — and use them against them. The task of the adult boy is to create a strong defence system, to minimise the risk of exposure.

The boy who was unable to express his feelings and has learnt early in his life that it is not okay to hold his mum's hand or sit on her lap and has learnt to suppress his vulnerable emotions. These small feelings then become stuck on the inside and can continue to dominate an adult man's life.

Unfelt emotions do not go away

Many grown men still feel like little boys on the inside. Some will think that others see or treat them like little boys.

How does it feel to be small? Most of us have forgotten what it felt like to be a child but from the vantage point of a child, everything is big. Adults look like giants, furniture is huge, buildings are enormous and the world is massive. Children can spend most of their time looking up and longing to grow up to see everything from the vantage point of big people. Being small can also be very frightening. A dog can be bigger. An adult could be hurtful. Children are powerless. They are physically weaker. They have less choice. They are reliant on others. They can feel defenceless.

If a child is not cared for, it is unlikely they will survive physically or emotionally. If a child felt their vulnerable feelings, it's unlikely they will want to feel those emotions ever again, as they are too painful and raw. Trust of others is formed in childhood. Can I trust that the big people in my life have my best interests at heart and will protect me? Will they listen to me? Do they love me? Children also learn about empathy. The child is entitled to ask questions: 'Do these big people seek to see the world from my perspective; do they care about how I see the world?

Peter, a forty-five-year-old man came to see me with anger issues. During our work together, he spoke about his childhood, how he had been fostered and been in care from a very young age. He had to move to a new home and family on a regular basis. To this day, he is unsure why this happened. He doesn't know his biological mother. Peter was a small man, he was also a bodybuilder and presents as a solid, rigid man with a hard exterior. He rarely smiles.

Peter did not receive unconditional love from appropriate adults and he was unable to feel secure and therefore develop a trusting relationship.

He learnt early on that in order to survive, he had to look after himself as it was clear that nobody else was going to do it for him. Any child brought up in this situation will experience a sense of loss and will commonly have a deficit of empathy. Peter's experience of being small is frightening, feeling constantly out of control and having no power over most of the major decisions that were impacting on his life.

My work with Peter initially meant creating a trustworthy relationship in which he could start to feel safe with another human being. I helped him to engage with the 'small' parts of himself that were ultimately still in control. Our work together enabled Peter to start to feel the feelings he had when he was little. These feelings were things he hadn't fully encountered; they were too overwhelming. He had been protecting himself from them.

When the man begins to embrace his inner 'smallness', paradoxically he will begin to feel bigger and more in control

---

When Peter was able to feel his inner pain, it was harder for others to provoke that small feeling inside. The psychological work that enabled his growth included embracing inner pain, embracing inner smallness, feeling one's powerlessness and taking the risk to enter into the frightening place of encountering vulnerable feelings. When this journey begins, the man will move from merely surviving to thriving. Ultimately, if we seek to deny the part of us that feels small or try to control 'going there' through avoidance techniques, defence systems and blaming others, then we will never be able to accept the part of us that is so desperate to be accepted, validated and cared for.

EMOTIONAL FITNESS TOOLBOX

1. Try to stop comparing yourself with others. When we compare, we come off worse. The person doing the comparing ends up in the 'less than' position, generating shame and making themselves feel smaller.

2. Think about 'Being Big' in your life — how do you strive to be big?

3. Observe your relationship with your penis — how does its rise and fall affect you and your feelings?

4. Make friends with your 'inner boy/girl'. This concept can often seem like psycho-babble. Many of my male clients end up working with the boy part of themselves, the inner-child who has not had his needs met and is, therefore, dominating his life. The inner boy needs to be given a safe place to be listened to, heard and cared for. The adult part of you is the best person to do this.

5. Invest in your smallness — talk to parents, siblings and old friends about your girl/ boyhood and keep a journal about childhood memories. Look at childhood photos and videos and listen to the child's unmet needs.

A TIP FOR WOMEN:

Try to refrain from shaming men about size. Yes, of course, be playful and tease them, but beware that many men are sensitive about this issue. If he has not done work on himself, you could trigger feelings of shame in him which are hard for him to deal with.

KEY #5

HE LONGS TO BE 'LOOKED AFTER' AND SO DOES SHE!

The majority of us enjoy being 'looked after' and cared for occasionally. We like it when others are thoughtful towards us, consider us and do things for us the way we like. The inner child part of us is still strong and we can often revert to that part of us, especially when we are struggling physically or psychologically. Many of us are also often driven by the ancient princess and prince (PAP) discourse that was introduced to us through fairytales, theme parks and Hollywood.

The PAP discourse can generate hidden and powerful longings which are learnt subconsciously through the influences mentioned above and from modelling expectations learnt from our family of origin (FOO). Within the PAP discourse, women may hold onto secret desires and longings to be swept off their feet by the knight in shining armour. They may wish to be protected and adored and dream of the romance of it all.

From the same discourse, men have been directed to find 'the one', the beautiful maiden who is waiting for him to appear. They will fall in love immediately and create a 'happily ever after'. These strong fantasies impact relationships on many levels, often with the couple unaware of their potency explored earlier in the book.

In my work with couples, some of the unspoken longings and expectations are made apparent when the relationship has fallen into functionality. The dissatisfaction leaks out through petty squabbles and deep frustration. When the relationship has moved away from romance due to children, work pressures, busyness and modern lifestyles the longing to be looked after may become very present, overwhelming and sometimes obsessive. The subtle expectations from the FOO and media influences can delay internal growth.

HAS HE LEFT HOME YET?

Leaving home psychologically is a hard thing to do. Growing up is painful. In the men's groups I facilitate one of the sessions is entitled, 'Have you left home yet?' This can often be the most challenging question and session for many. Most men have, of course, physically left home but unfortunately, many more have yet to psychologically leave home. They still desire to be mothered and looked after.

In relationships, the uncut umbilical cord can cause ongoing conflicts between a man and his partner. His loyalty may remain with his mother at the expense of his relationship. These men may be the hard, macho, top of the pile men and would never be seen as a 'mummy's boy' externally, but internally the strong bond and link has never been adjusted with regard to his new family, his adult life and status.

Until the adult male can psychologically leave home, he will remain a boy. To move to manhood, he will need to cut the psychological umbilical cord

---

THE MIDLIFE CRISIS

A midlife crisis is not inevitable but it will be if a man never leaves home psychologically. The discontentment and unmet needs felt in his earlier life will come back with vengeance often leaving men swamped in obsessive and powerful feelings.

The transition from the first to the second half of life leads to a period of reflection on the past including regrets and preparing body and mind for the next phase of life. The phrase, 'You only live once' is flashed in neon lights wherever you look and feelings, needs, and wants become alive and difficult to ignore.

The core question asked at this stage of life is this: 'Have my basic needs been met?' The second question to the self is: 'How do I get my unmet needs/desires met?

Some of the following questions may also be asked: Do I get enough attention? Is it the right kind of attention? How do I receive affirmation? Am I really known? What does my body still yearn for? Have I had enough sex? Do I feel connected to other people? Do I fully know others? What makes me fully alive? Am I happy? Has my life been fulfilling so far? What am I missing? Would anyone really miss me? Who am I? Am I presenting my true self or am I living a lie? Do I actually like the person I live with? What can I change that will give me a greater sense of at-one-ness?

These are deep and possibly dangerous questions which could generate massive lifestyle changes. Responses to these questions can cause people to do things they would never have imagined themselves doing. If this middle passage is not traversed with awareness, then it can often turn into a midlife crisis in which people's lives are disrupted with often shocking consequences.

The midlife crisis can lead some to revert to the past, seeking to relive their youth and do the things they feel they missed out on. For men, this stage in life can often lead to sexual liaisons and affairs with younger women or it might include risky activities and speed, usually involving a motorbike or sports car. The clichéd image of a man in his 50s or 60s with a motorbike and a younger girlfriend is often accurate.

Instead of navigating this important life stage and deciding to reach for a new maturity and awareness, many men become stuck in the past and on a loop of doing more of the same external thing that they feel will bring happiness. The second half of life invites us to explore what is inside of us, to focus on our spiritual and emotional growth, to develop inner beauty, depth and wisdom.

When we meet the second half of life with psychological awareness the answers to life's challenges will often be found internally rather than externally. Unfortunately, society has become so consumed with the external, with appearance, beauty, the cult of youth and external experience that few take the path described in Frost's poem and Peck's book, 'The road less travelled'.

THE MOTHER AND THE WHORE

There is a deep part in most men which is about being cared for and nurtured. They long to be cared for by a loving, warm woman. Men still desire to be mothered and nurtured by the homemaker with her 'natural' ability to take care of her man's physical needs. The old proverb that says 'The way to a man's heart is through his stomach' clearly holds true. The table where families meet for meals is often the communal heart of the home, with wholesome homemade food emerging from the traditionally female-run kitchen.

If a man's wife/partner can cook good food like his mother and provide for his physical needs, then she will have his love. Almost as if his wife is as good a cook as his biological mother then his wife will be a worthy replacement, after all, she knows what he likes. When the man has yet to leave home psychologically, he can often cling onto what has gone before: 'Mother knows what I like'. This stance is backward looking and can ruin his present relationship if he is unaware of it. His unspoken or unconscious expectations mean that he expects his partner to know exactly what he likes and to magically know what he is thinking.

Some men will protest at the above paragraph, suggesting that modern men have moved on from this antiquated view and practice. It is right that modern families do share domestic tasks much more. However, even when both adults are working full-time, the female will still do 75% of the domestic chores. The woman will fulfil the majority of the needs of the children including school issues, buying clothes, helping with homework, and arranging social engagements.

I regularly hear issues very similar to these when young couples come to my clinic. The typical situation goes as follows: the female returns from a busy day at work, having just picked up the children and prepared food. The male partner returns home from work and is angry that the house is a tip and that he isn't met with a smile and a cup of tea. Instead of helping, the man will then duck out of responsibilities. He will have time to himself, have a bath, watch TV or do some work.

Men and fathers are clearly more engaged with the family than they used to be, but I have heard the above story from young couples on numerous occasions. I think the deep-set expectations have to be addressed to generate fulfilled relationships. In my experience, the female is still often viewed as the 'Great mother and nurturer' and 'Daddy's day-care' is open inconsistently. Mothers will inevitably feel put-upon and exhausted if the man does not help. On top of this, the man also wants the woman to look after him sexually. He longs for the whore or sex goddess who will instinctively know how to please him sexually.

A common desire for men is that women are always available for sex. The meta sexual fantasy is that she will take total care of him in the kitchen.The mother and whore become one. He fantasises that she will be preparing food while dressed in lingerie and will always be ready to provide for his physical comforts

Sexual fantasies and desire are quite complex. Psychology surrounding power is often at work. Even the fact that men are turned on by women dressed in frilly, soft lingerie. Dressed like a little girl surely must create pause for thought. Why does this turn men on? Is it because he feels he can 'take care' of her?

Often men want to be sexually 'looked after' by a woman who initiates and fulfils his desires. One of the reasons some men want riskier sex or sex with a prostitute is that she will be willing to do what he wants. She will know what to do. His inner expectations will be met and it is ultimately thrilling.

If food is the way to a man's heart, is sex the way to hold onto his presence?

The whore is always available for sex. She wants it and initiates it. The attraction of prostitutes and the message of porn, is that women are always available for sex and will be ready to please men in any way the man wants. Perhaps, this longing for gratification is connected to the child and the inner boy's longing for his mother to meet his needs, to love him in all ways, after all, 'Mother knows best'.

The book called 'The Truth — an uncomfortable book about relationships' is a fascinating read regarding men's obsession with sex. The reason this book is especially significant regarding sex is that the author Neil Strauss also authored 'The Game' where he advocates freedom and sex and teaches men how to pick up lots of women. In 'The Truth', Strauss describes his personal journey away from addiction to sex and towards love. He discusses his therapeutic discoveries about the roots of his constant need for sex connecting it to unmet needs in his relationship with his mother. Strauss writes:

> *'I was never actually pursuing sexual freedom. I was pursuing control, power, and self-worth. I was either acting like my mom or making someone into my mom. Rarely was I actually myself. Because, as I witnessed on ecstasy, the feeling that I'm not acceptable as I am is so fucking overwhelming that I'm terrified to let go and just be myself with anyone.'*[38]

In this book, Strauss addresses his relationship with his inner boy and moves away from his sex games and towards intimacy and connection. This man has had sex with hundreds of women and with several at the same time. Yet, his massive appetite for sex left him unfulfilled, unhappy and empty. Fortunately, he had the courage to take responsibility for his life and was willing to do the painful work becoming aware of his inner needs and to feel his feelings.

DO MEN SECRETLY FEAR THE POWER OF WOMEN?

I wonder if men unconsciously fear women or as described by Strauss, are acting out unresolved issues with their mothers.

In ancient times it wasn't the male god that was worshipped, it was the female goddess. Before medical knowledge and understanding about genealogy, tribes were in awe of the women's changing body and the miracle of her giving birth to another human. The woman was the life-giver. She created life and was the great nurturer. Apart from carrying new life, she was also able to stand an immense amount of pain.

Are men secretly in awe of women and in some way fear her inner power and strength and have responded by generationally subjecting her? Many men still regard women as the 'weaker' sex and have sought to take her power, reduce her to a second-class citizen and imprison her in the home.

It's only in the last century that women have begun to be more empowered but the old attitudes often remain. In the last hundred years, women have gained the vote, received more equality and entered the workplace in increasing numbers. There is still a long way to go, with regular setbacks and backlashes from men who feel emasculated.

Fact: all men come from women

As mentioned in my discussion on shame, boys and men often feel a sense of loss in relation to their mother, but the yearning is still there perhaps played out in unhealthy and unfulfilled ways. Is there a part of the man that is always desiring to reconnect with the mother and the feminine and is this the desire some men seek to fulfil through cross-dressing, transvestism and the culturally accepted British pastime of pantomime?

As Mick Jagger once said: 'British men don't need much persuading to dress up as women.' Perhaps this is a way for men to get in touch with a lost part of themselves that the dominant culture has prevented. These are questions, not assertions but there is no doubt in my mind that men have broken off a part of themselves and for the rest of their lives are often seeking to reconnect with this loss in whatever way they can.

For men to move from the position of equalising intimacy with sex, it will be important for him to consider his relationship with his mother and his views and treatment of women.

MAN FLU IS REAL

If there is one thing men are often jibed about, it is 'Man flu'. This term describes how men can fake illness and act a little pathetic as a way to be looked after by their partner. Man flu allows men to be given extra attention. It is a good excuse for a while to do nothing.

Perhaps 'Man Flu' is the way that the 'little boy' can receive sympathy, comfort and attention. He can feel he is allowed to be looked after. After all, being saddled with the job of being the provider and protector is a heavy psychological burden. Men are often caught in the trap of having to be tough and strong and can struggle to have the vocabulary to express their needs and so these feelings may emerge and be expressed through physical affirmation and passion.

'Man flu' has become a common cultural term used to describe a man being a bit ineffective and pathetic. His partner is unconvinced about the severity of his illness: 'he isn't really ill!' However, according to recent research, 'Man Flu' isn't a myth, it is in fact real.

Apparently, men get sick more often, because they don't have the sex hormones which boost women's immune systems. Oestrogen helps fight off respiratory infections according to a research team from Harvard University, who experimented with female and male mice. You may be thinking that the research team were all male but that wasn't the case.

FLU IS REAL

I have only experienced flu once in my lifetime. It was debilitating and horrible. It included headaches, fatigue, muscle ache, head cold and I was totally zapped of energy. I was bedbound for at least a week, then indoors for another week. Then it took another two to four weeks to get back normal energy.

Having experienced this virus, my flu fascist antennae will raise its head when I hear people dismissing the illness. When I hear most people describe flu, what I think most of them mean is that they have contracted the 'common cold' and I, of course, need to put them right.

THE ROOTS OF 'MAN FLU' MOCKING

You may be reading this and wondering why I am writing about 'Man Flu'. My point is mainly about how men have been conditioned to look after themselves. Self-reliance, as previously mentioned, is a core way for men to take care of themselves.

Men will feel safe to ask for help and be reliant on others when the body has broken bones, when blood flows, or an illness is life-threatening

---

An illness that is not externally obvious can be seen as 'fake' by others. The man may risk exposure to shame. When mental or emotional health is considered in this context, men may struggle to recognise their need for support and find it incredibly hard to ask for help, due to the man rules.

Contrast this kind of 'weak' man with the 'strong, silent wilderness man', who will seek solitude and isolation and enhance the self-reliant status of masculinity. This way of being relies on the independent spirit, but it increases the walls of self-denial and keeps the weaknesses of 'neediness', 'tenderness' and 'touch' at bay. Distance from the 'softness' of women is the only way to preserve that masculine edge.

I wonder if 'man flu' has become a parody which men and women have subconsciously agreed and accepted, in order to enable men to manage feeling unwell when it is not a life-threatening situation. Man flu allows the tough and strong man to 'act pathetic', be needy and come across like a little boy who needs to be looked after. Most men will know about 'man flu' and hence it is normalised and universally mocked — ultimately this helps to disperse the shame that men feel.

There is a root cause to man flu and this is linked to selfishness. Within the male rule of self-reliance, men have become experienced at getting their perceived needs met. They have learnt to look after themselves. They can also play 'the boy' to be looked after. Due to the power of self-reliance, many men struggle to look after others. If men hold onto the coping skill of self-reliance in relationships then it will cause relational difficulties. Some men can come down with man flu to avoid domestic chores or shirk some difficult task.

However, few men will allow man flu to prevent them from doing things they really want to do, like their favourite sport or hobby or spending time in the pub with their mates. Their partner may be very accommodating to this lifestyle because she feels she has no option. An accommodating attitude may though be covering up a dissatisfaction about the roles and responsibilities they have adopted.

Men, it is time to learn to take care of yourself and others

MANY MEN SHIRK WORK AT HOME

As mentioned earlier in this chapter, the woman in a relationship will often do most of the domestic chores and childcare. Some men will never even consider children's clothing, their schooling, arranging play dates with friends, presents for parties or worrying about their child's overall wellbeing. Many will not consider doing more for their children.

When it comes to parents adjusting their working schedule to accommodate childcare, men tend to think the female will adjust her working patterns. When men do look after their children, they can sometimes think they are doing the mother a favour and feel like a superhero.

Some men refer to taking care of their own children as 'Daddy day-care'. They like to be applauded by others when seen in public looking after their children, almost as if they are superheroes!

On one occasion, I took my young children food shopping. Whilst packing my bags, I was told that I was being a great babysitter. I was being praised for taking care of my children, as if I was doing my wife and children a favour, as if this was an unusual event.

Even though male celebrity chefs dominate cooking programmes on television, it is still the case that women will do the majority of the home cooking and food shopping. Doing household chores is something that many women take care of. Personally, I don't mind cleaning, but I don't do much of it and my wife will often have to ask/remind me to do it. I will only get the hoover out when the mess becomes strikingly obvious. I am not sure that women like cleaning either, but they will end up doing it because they cannot cope with the mess any longer. Some people employ a cleaner to overcome this problem. This solves some of these problems, but many of the relational arguments can be about a man's lack of engagement with housework.

When the above is taking into consideration and men then come down with 'the flu', it is easy to identify a lack of female sympathy. Women may feel that men are shirking or faking illness, because it appears to come on when they are relaxed; so it can appear at weekends or when they are on holiday. Can you see the link? Resentment and anger can emerge as his wife/partner feels she is taken for granted, that she is treated as the great mother. Not only does she have to maintain a full-time job, look after the children and do all the housework, now she is expected to look after her 'sick' male partner. The saying has evolved: 'It's like having three children to look after.'

MEN AND SELF-CARE

Men traditionally are not good at self-care. They often think they are indestructible and should not show any sign of weakness, which is of course how mental illness is then also perceived. As I have mentioned previously, many men are not in tune with their bodies. They fail to listen to the signs of physical and mental illness before a problem becomes more serious.

Men often put off going to the doctor due to multiple reasons and fail to listen to the signs of physical and mental illness before a problem becomes more serious. A client was telling me about a male friend who was aware he had an odd lump in his throat and yet he ignored it and refused to go to the doctor. Eventually, he became aware of other unusual symptoms and with encouragement from his family went to get medical help. By the time he got help, the cancer had spread from his throat to other parts of his body.

Often this avoidant behaviour is about men being afraid of the unknown, using the old coping strategy of ignoring things and hoping they will disappear. Due to the man's lack of self-care and his inaction, his whole family and friends were now involved in caring for him and often carrying his emotional pain. Often, women will feel they need to step in and arrange an appointment with the GP or counsellor as a way of looking after themselves and the relationship.

Men, it's time to take care of yourselves! Stop relying on the old survival skill of denial, avoidance and isolation. Stop expecting others to carry your emotional baggage and look after your own emotional needs. It is time to stop expecting others to look after your physical and social needs.

Only when men begin to take care of themselves will they be able to finally take care of others, their children, their partners and their friends.

It is time to stop relying on your mother, your wife and your daughters to look after you; it is time for you to grow up

---

Mothers, you need to let your sons go and stop doing everything for them. Wives and partners encourage him to take responsibility for relational growth, emotional growth and social engagements. Refuse to collude with the PAP discourse and seek to challenge the unspoken expectations. Stop doing everything for him. Men, it is time for you to finally grow up and psychologically leave home.

EMOTIONAL FITNESS TOOLBOX

1. Develop self-care. Do one-minute check-ins throughout the day. Listen to your inner chatter. Listen to your body.

2. Are you too busy? What is your work/life balance like? Make a timetable and balance up the hours you spend at work, time with your partner and family, the time you devote to leisure and the time you spend doing chores around the house.

3. Health check — book in a health check with your GP and book in with a counsellor for an emotional MOT.

4. Arrange to talk to your partner about unspoken expectations and roles. Stop assuming that s/he knows your needs. Begin to talk about your sex life and expectations. By suggesting this to your partner and taking some responsibility for your relationship, I can guarantee this one act will improve your relationship.

5. Leave home psychologically by doing some work to unpick the influences your parents have/had over you. What are your expectations of him/her? Practise taking responsibility for your needs and verbalise them to your partner. Remember s/he is not your parent!

KEY #6

MEN'S VULNERABLE FEELINGS ARE EXPRESSED THROUGH ANGER

'Anyone can become angry — that is easy,
but to be angry with the right person at the right time
and for the right purpose and in the right way —
that is not within everyone's power and that is not easy.'

— ARISTOTLE[39]

Aristotle's quote is a brilliant description of emotional fitness. Anger is a normal and important emotion and when expressed healthily is an essential part of emotional fitness. However, in our society, many people are struggling to manage and understand their anger with little awareness. They are out of control in how they express their anger; it will come out in sudden and dramatic bursts, through aggressive behaviour and violence. Anger is seen as a negative and destructive emotion, so an unhealthy discourse has arisen around it.

Some psychologists are intent on generating an emotional dualism — they want a hierarchy of positive and negative emotions. The 'happiness' project promotes helping us to generate habits, people, and activities that make us happier. Of course, we all would like to be happy. But we cannot experience happiness without also experiencing sadness, disappointment and hurt. Focusing on experiencing one emotion will actually reduce emotional fitness.

It can generate an emotional fascism in which people expressing other emotions can be seen as negative influences and to be rooted out of one's life. Happiness can actually be expressed in an unhealthy way and may appear insincere or inauthentic. In my view, emotions are neither positive nor negative, they just are. To be fully human, we need to be able to experience, feel and express the full spectrum of emotions.

There are NO negative emotions

Anger gets a bad press. This is because of its external expression, often associated with aggression. It has become an emotion that cannot be expressed. Many people will associate anger and aggression as the same thing. There are, however, many ways of expressing anger though more commonly it seeps out, which can often be more dangerous than external aggressiveness.

Fritz Pearls once said the root of aggression is to go out, to move and to meet the other. To 'aggress' is in fact, a positive force that moves us to connect and make contact with the other. It propels us out of our aloneness in order to seek to be touched and to touch, which is a positive thing for everybody.

BASIC SURVIVAL SKILLS

Many people in the world spend the majority of their time physically surviving by finding and fetching water each day, making fire, finding food, cooking and eating. They then continue with the same routine the next day.

Bear Grylls created a TV programme called 'The Island' where he leaves a group of people on an isolated island. Their one and only challenge is to survive. These programmes show how their daily life is consumed by the need for water, fire, food and shelter. 'First world' problems like appearance, nice smelling bodies and social networking are quickly forgotten. It's not long before group conflict emerges. Keeping their bodies fuelled and safe becomes the overriding concern and driver.

On one programme, celebrities were introduced to the island. It became apparent, very soon, bodies that looked great were useless in this situation. A rugby player with a toned and muscular torso quickly found himself becoming lethargic, due to a lack of body fat. He had to leave the island very early in order to survive. The people whose bodies had more fat reserves were able to maintain physical energy for longer.

Everyone is hardwired with an internal, natural defence system which is programmed to keep us safe. When one lives in a world of basic physical survival, the instinct is to move our bodies when there is a perceived threat. There is no time to think or to analyse the threat. We just naturally act and our brain directs the body to defend itself through either fight, flight, freeze or appease. When we are physically threatened, the instinctive reaction is to defend through our default position. Depending on the situation, your instinct may be to run.

My default survival strategy is definitely to move away. I am vigilant of situations I think might be threatening and keep away. I am not a fighter and don't have confidence in my fighting abilities. I would definitely see flight as my first choice but if I needed to protect my family then, of course, I would try and fight.

Freezing is not such an obvious defence tactic, but it can equally be a good strategy to employ when danger threatens. In the wild, some animals will become totally still while camouflaging themselves. They will be motionless, waiting until the potential attacker has passed them by. Likewise, during a threatening situation such as encountering a spree killer who is shooting people indiscriminately, playing dead could be the very best protective strategy.

Appeasement is another way of dealing with imminent danger, which may take the form of offering the attacker something in order to save one's life. This might include gifts, sex or giving some sort of power away.

Abraham Maslow was an eminent psychologist who created the famous 'hierarchy of needs'. He emphasised the importance of basic needs being met: shelter, warmth and food come first. Maslow highlighted the importance of certain needs being met before one could focus on 'higher' needs such as socialising and education.

In our modern world, many of us no longer have to worry about finding food, water and making fire and hence more time can go into meeting 'higher' needs. Maslow's original 'hierarchy of needs' has been given a modern twist (see image below) with modern needs for survival added. Portable devices such as smartphones have become a huge part of our daily lives and some people struggle to live without them.

'I can't live without my phone.'

— A FEMALE TEENAGER CLIENT

Screen addiction is becoming a real concern in contemporary society. Recent data has shown how often and how long we all spend looking at our smartphones and other screens. A charged battery and access to WIFI becomes a pseudo important survival need. When my boys were little and we were in the car on a long journey, we often used to hear the classic cry of 'are we there yet?'

These days before we leave on a trip, the first items to be packed are screens, chargers and options to charge the battery. Checking if our destination has WIFI access could make the kids more enthusiastic about the holiday. Now in the car, what we hear is 'Can I just finish my game!' For our family, holidays are an important time to have a break from screens, so we often camp and try and find places where the internet connection is weak. This allows us to be more connected to each other and spend more time outside and being active.

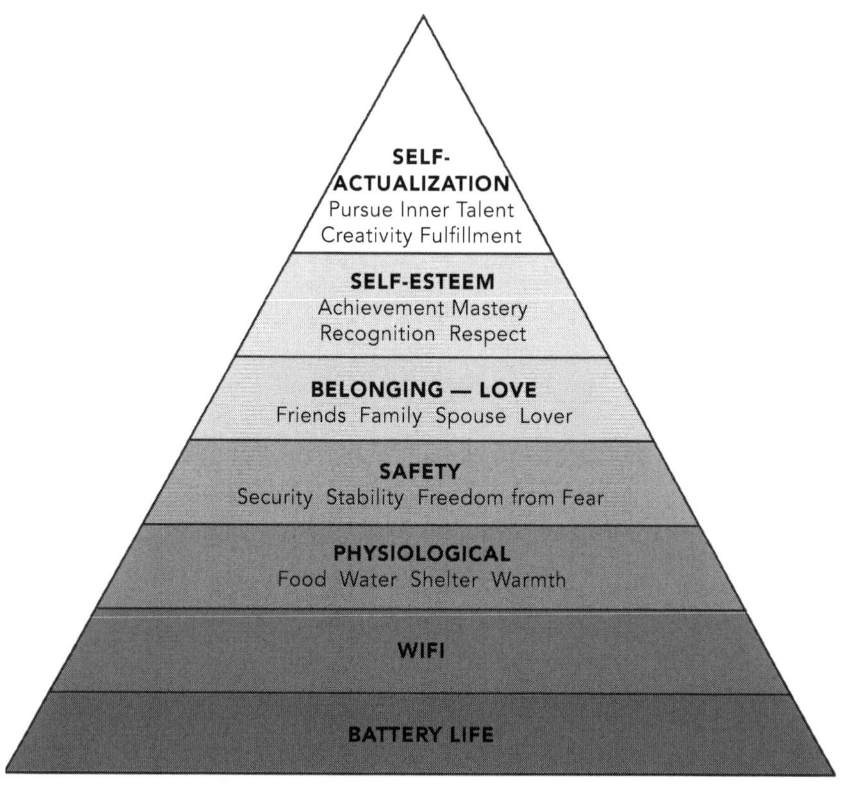

MOVING FROM SURVIVING TO THRIVING

When basic survival needs are met and the individual experiences stability, security and confidence, then he or she can start to move from merely surviving to thriving. For the majority of us living in materially wealthy countries, natural survival instincts will kick in when facing a physical threat. For many people, the ability to emotionally survive when psychologically threatened remains instinctive, with the inability to choose an emotional response.

When one feels under emotional threat in terms of feelings exposed or vulnerable or ultimately at risk, the instinctive emotional survival mechanism called anger will often kick in to defend emotional fragility. It may not always look like anger but subtle techniques are developed, including concealing, denying or projecting anger.

We develop our emotional survival skills very early in life. Children are amazing at physically surviving and can do this even within very abusive, chaotic and dysfunctional home situations. However, in doing this, they often have to shut down or suppress parts of themselves. Their vulnerable emotions are the key ones to protect. If they allow themselves to feel their vulnerable emotions, they would lose the resilience to survive.

Adults often perpetuate the myth that children are amazingly resilience and can cope with difficult situations. Children are actually very good at adapting to difficult situations, due to the physical survival instinct, but in so doing have to let go of feeling and expressing their vulnerable feelings.

Carl Rogers (creator of Person Centred therapy) suggested that children learn 'conditions of worth'. This means children will work out how to act appropriately to stand the best chance of receiving their carer's love and acceptance. The child will identify that to be loved and accepted, she or he will have to abide by certain rules, which could include the following:

1. Don't get angry/don't shout
2. Always leave a clean plate
3. Only talk when you are spoken to
4. Always say 'please' and 'thank you'
5. Don't become unwell
6. Do not be sad or cry

Abiding by these conditions without any expression of emotion, will eventually create emotional survival skills and result in suppressing true feelings as the child feels unaccepted in an unsafe environment. The message children have internalised is that they need to hide a part of themselves or restrict certain emotions to meet their need to be loved. The unexpressed feelings are left to reside inside them and need to be controlled and managed as a way of protecting the vulnerable, authentic self.

If the child is unable to suppress his/her emotions, the feelings might emerge as anger. The child may then be diagnosed with an anger management 'disorder' and will be sent to get treatment.

I work with many children and teenagers referred to me in order to sort out their anger. One such boy, let's call him Alex, was displaying aggressive behaviour at home and at school. Alex is an intelligent and articulate ten-year-old boy and was the oldest of three siblings. When he came to see me, he had moved from another country and was now living in the UK. He was now attending his second school. Alex's behaviour included violent rages at other students, displaying unusual physical behaviours including head banging. He was unafraid to question or 'speak back' to authority figures, including head teachers. His behaviour at home was also becoming more difficult.

His parents were becoming concerned about his behaviour and Alex arrived for a session with his father. During the first session, Alex began to describe his angry outbursts, continually checking how Dad was responding to what he was saying. Whilst describing his anger he began to talk about his sadness and with tears in his eyes said to his Dad, 'I bet you didn't know that about me, did you?' Alex then described how, after an incident at school, he felt sad and to stop himself from crying, he banged his head against a wall.

As I got to know Alex, I felt that his rage and difficult behaviour were coming from his emotional defence system. His anger was one way of him generating some power in his life and expressing his more vulnerable feelings. I wondered if in the busyness and stress in his family, he had learnt that unhappiness was not acceptable. Alex did not feel safe enough to express his powerful feelings and therefore they seeped out. I knew Alex needed to be heard and understood; if it didn't happen, I would expect the difficult behaviour would continue. His unmet needs and expression of the right feelings needed to be welcomed and encouraged.

When the child becomes an adult, the inner child still carries these old conditions of worth and may still react or behave in the same way as she/he did as a child. These inner emotions can turn into emotional monsters, becoming more difficult to contain with the increased threat of being released. The fear of 'lifting the lid' and 'opening a can of worms' describes how uncomfortable feelings are suppressed and many will take the option of leaving them where they are. The lid is kept firmly screwed on due to the emotional myth and fear that if these feelings are released, then the person may lose control.

The BIG feelings — the ones we fear the most — are in fact the feelings which make us feel the smallest

---

The powerful feelings, the ones we find hard to express are the feelings that 'make us feel small' like sadness, helplessness, hurt, feeling powerless, fear and shame. These are the vulnerable emotions or as many men have been told, the weak emotions!

ANGER IS OUR EMOTIONAL DEFENCE SYSTEM

Emotional danger emerges when we feel under threat. A vulnerable emotion could be exposed; at this point, anger kicks in as a basic survival instinct.

Anger is an emotional defence system. It is activated when anything we encounter threatens to penetrate the person's vulnerable emotions

---

Anger becomes the emotional defence system to protect the organism from feeling or exposing vulnerable feelings that could then open the gate for further threats. The defence system may operate in several different ways but could include responding with certain behaviours in order to get unmet needs met.

For men, the default emotion is often anger

Earlier in this book, I suggested that men's default emotion was often anger. I illustrated this with a picture of how the typical emotional grid would look. Due to male conditioning through the male code, men's emotional spectrum has been severely reduced. This has left many men blinded by anger, they are unable to see a bigger spectrum of emotion and expression because their default state is one of anger.

Men dare not express their vulnerable emotions out of fear of being accused of weakness and smallness, hence these feelings have been hidden and disguised. Anger then turns into a monster.

Men have been conditioned to protect their inner fragility by employing anger as their emotional security guard

---

Men have heard and learnt that 'Big Boys' don't cry. They eventually lose touch with their inner sadness. They lose the ability to recognise sadness and eventually their tear ducts dry up. Many men will do anything to prevent themselves being seen as soft and wet.

Emitting moisture in an uncontrolled way is shameful, unless it is in the form of urine, sweat or semen

---

Having no way of expressing the flow of sadness restricts the healing potency of this normal emotion. Men can find themselves weeping in the dark when alone but less so in public. My learning for the past fifteen years has been relearning how to cry. I have probably wept more alone and in public than in the previous forty years. I have cried in the arms of my son, my friends and my wife. I have heaved sobs of tears in the safety of my men's group and it has felt so healing.

Men are bombarded with messages that they should be tough and strong. They have learnt to swallow hard and suck the fear in, by regularly seeking to live by the message of 'show no fear' which constantly rings in their ears. Men have been taught to work hard against revealing any 'weakness' and to prove themselves by partaking in extreme and risky behaviours, sports and pursuits. However, losing touch with anxiety and fear is dangerous as it is our natural warning system against threats. To constantly override fear can have dire consequences, with men literally pushing themselves over the edge.

Men have even had to contain happiness. Giggling or showing joy and exhilaration can be perceived as a bit childish or 'girly' and ultimately soft. As mentioned previously, this kind of joy is only allowed to be emoted when your team scores. But generally, the poker face of men doesn't move unless it is at another man's expense.

Anger has become like an oversized muscle similar to a sportsman preparing his body for a particular sport and building certain muscles. For instance, a road cyclist will develop very strong legs and yet his upper body is skinny, with little muscle. To be emotionally fit, men will need to exercise the full range of emotional muscles in order to be more balanced and healthier.

Men's default emotional grid is a good example of how anger is perceived. It is the big emotion and it is extremely powerful. When there is a chance of feeling small, then the big emotion of anger steps in to take charge. Often the best form of defence is offence.

KAPOW! — Anger is the protector of small fragile emotions

Another way to explain this is to talk about the small inner boy men have inside them. When his 'boy' feels under threat or his needs remain unmet, then the big part of himself defends the boy from hurt and pain. It is important to remember the roots of anger are a sense of powerlessness, feeling out of control and feeling trapped.

THE FIVE ANGER STYLES AND HOW THESE IMPACT ON RELATIONSHIPS

I've identified five anger styles. Describing these styles to clients provides them with the knowledge to have a clearer understanding of their anger. This leads to greater awareness and the possibility of change. Expressing anger in a certain style is a choice. It may not feel that way and is often unconscious but the reason I say it is a choice, is that men and, of course, women will display different anger styles depending on the environment and the person involved. I'm going to describe these styles in a little more detail below.

THE FIVE ANGER STYLES

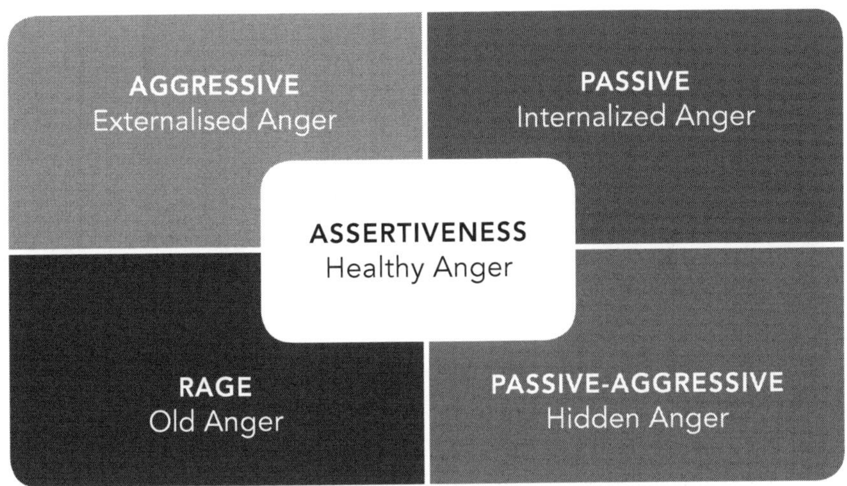

1. Aggressive — Externalised anger

When people think of anger, most associate it with externalised or aggressive anger. This state of anger flows outward and is released into the world. We may have met people who always appear to be angry about something. They act defensively and will be quick to fire a few rounds at anyone they don't like.

Being externally angry regularly is not healthy and this pent up, explosive anger not only pushes people away but the person expressing anger ends up absorbing a huge amount of energy. The person who is aggressive feels the world is out to get them. They have an underlying sense that something is being done to them.

The 'Aggressive' has two mottos for life:
'the best form of defence is attack' and 'it's not fair'

The aggressive feels that life owes them something and when it doesn't come their way, they will have to fight for it or blame the other. Expressing anger in this way, however, could be seen as having some health benefits with a 'better out than in' approach. Anger is indeed a powerful feeling and it moves us towards motions and therefore expressing E-Motion.

Physical movement can in some way stop us from getting stuck. There is no doubt that moving our body through running or some other activity can help disperse the intensity of this difficult emotion. For many years, the advice for angry young men has been to exercise it through sport, boxing or on the football terraces. Sport is very important for a lot of men. It's a way of channelling energy, anger and aggression.

But this is only part of the story and fails to help the aggressive to fully move it and release it. The energy could end up being moved in unhealthy ways by hurting oneself and others. Many parents ask me if I think boxing will help their sons to release their anger. I usually tell them that boxing will not help, in fact it may make it worse. The core problem is that it teaches boys and men to store up, contain and carry anger until it can be released in a designated area. The problem with 'releasing' anger out of context is that it gives little awareness to the triggers of the anger and thus leaves the aggressive feeling powerless to harness or understand their anger.

The danger of externalised anger is that it tends to shift the pain and the intense feelings onto others. Aggressive people need to be seen, heard and felt often through violence. When this kind of anger gets out of control it can lead to harming others emotionally and physically with the worst-case scenario ending in murder.

Your anger is no one else's fault

Ultimately, aggressive anger is the child's tantrum. It is a cry for attention. This kind of anger brings much attention and connection to the person. It is the cry of the inner child's unmet needs and is effectively saying 'I am not coping' and 'You are not meeting my expectations'.

SHOUT — AN ANGER AWARENESS PROGRAMME

I have written and facilitated an anger awareness programme called SHOUT. It is for men from all walks of life. It has been running since 2004. On the advertising, I describe the programme as 'anger management' but I'll be honest — I am not very interested in managing anger. The SHOUT programme creates a safe environment for men to become aware of the roots of anger and it provides a space for them to talk about their feelings in relation to anger. SHOUT is based on the following five concepts:

1. Exploring and developing masculinity
2. Developing emotional fitness
3. Developing body awareness
4. Psycho-educational input in relation to the psychology of anger
5. Practise and rehearsal

The programme includes a lot of physical interaction, movement, discussion, expression of vulnerable feelings, anger release work and very little paper-based work. In my view, there is nothing wrong with getting your anger out, as long as it doesn't hurt others or yourself. I personally actually enjoy the movement of shouting but I have to take responsibility for how and where I exercise it and how I express it.

If moving anger externally enables you to be aware of your anger and the roots, then it is healthy. In some of my work with clients, I may use voice work or anger release work through use of a punch bag or a bat and a pillow. Bodywork is important to help men become more in tune with their bodies. It helps them to listen to its movements, sensations and pain and then respond to this information in a healthy way.

2. Passive — Internalised anger

Passive anger expression is the polar opposite of the aggressive with the natural response being 'flight' and to move away from the anger, silently absorbing it. Classically this state or style of anger is directed inside, in which the person turns anger against himself or herself. They end up eventually, hurting themselves. The passive internalises the anger and believes he/she is the problem and the inner discourse sounds like this 'It is my fault and I am the problem.'

Personally, passive anger expression is my default style of anger. When I was a child, my survival skill was to please others by agreeing with them or appeasing them. By acting in this way, I thought I would be liked and accepted. My emotional work on this issue has led me to explore my shame, which has often kept me living inside my own head.

As a boy, I can remember I would always be vigilant to an external attack. This often meant I would seek to be invisible. This technique or survival strategy has caused me numerous problems in later life, contributing to a 'poor me' and 'it's not fair' script and the feeling that I have lacked the attention I deserve. My survival technique prevented painful feelings or exposure, but it left me living much of my world internally, while seeing externally motivated people move on. My way of meeting the world was reinforced by a certain theology I encountered as a boy within the Christian Strict Baptist tradition.

Authentic emotional expression was normally frowned upon. Expression of Anger was generally kept under wraps

---

It was generally perceived that anger was a sin or wrong, although this teaching was not actually based on good theology. I think this particular code was more about maintaining control of emotions and therefore needing to suppress rather than risk externalising them. As a boy and young man, I was committed to a muscular or masochistic kind of spirituality, in which I felt I needed to prove my spiritual maturity and credentials by suppressing any 'worldly' desires.

One particular text which supported my shame and aligned with my internal script was a text credited to Jesus; 'Deny yourself, take up your cross and follow me'. What I understood by this as it was reinforced by Baptist teaching was that I should deny myself pleasure, distrust self, and declare war on myself. This did a lot of damage to my fragile ego, leading to me being a boy and a man who at his core felt deeply shamed and disconnected to self. This kind of theology connected to conditions of worth left me with a survival skill that hindered my growth. I spent decades unlearning this faulty theology and seeking to unravel a warped sense of self.

Passive people internalise their anger and live in fear of upsetting others. They spend a lot of time and energy appeasing others and taking the blame. Passives suppress or suck down their anger fearing to speak it. My anger could be seen as it warmed up my body and illuminated my face through blushing leading to shaming.

Passive anger internalises emotion causing internal damage. It is exaggerated through negative and destructive self-talk

---

All of us engage in an internal dialogue that is perfectly natural and healthy. What passives have to work on is developing the discipline of 'capturing' negative self-talk and replacing it with positive self-talk and gratitude. Learning to be kind to yourself and developing self-compassion are incredibly important. Learning self-compassion and letting the inner self off the hook is an important practice to prevent internalising harmful anger.

Passives self-harm physically, which can show itself through neglecting themselves or through actual physical self-harm in all its guises from punching walls, cutting and pushing their bodies to extremes. The extreme end of the spectrum of this kind of anger is of course suicide. Passive anger can also contribute to all sorts of physical ailments and mental health problems including IBS, cancer, immune disorders, migraines, chronic back issues, anxiety, depression and other emotional or mental health disorders.

3. Passive-aggressive — Hidden anger or indirect anger

We are all fairly experienced at being passive-aggressive. Passive-aggressive anger is subtle and sneaky and seeps out through the body and through the mouth, hoping not to be noticed. It is indirect and delivered incognito seeking to ask the receiver to take responsibility for the projected anger. It is a very difficult anger to identify and capture and can feel like an invisible attack. The receiver can feel that something has just happened to them but is left unsure about what happened or where the attack came from. This kind of anger expression is often endemic and the perpetrator is often unaware of what they are doing.

If it is identified and named the deliverer will expect the receiver to take responsibility for it by responding with things like, 'Can't you take a laugh' or 'lighten up'. Women can often be told to 'smile, it might never happen' by men who would like women to respond to them in a certain way and is an expression of indirect anger. A passive-aggressive is unwilling to directly express his/her anger. They secretly want the other to feel their anger and even express their anger for them. When the other expresses the anger, the passive-aggressive then blames them for being angry!

The root of passive-aggressive anger is a refusal by the sender to take responsibility for their emotion. They subtly invite someone else to feel it, receive it and express it for them

---

PASSIVE-AGGRESSIVE ANGER CAN BE EXPRESSED IN DIFFERENT WAYS:

- **NON-COMMUNICATION** — when there is something problematic to discuss.
- **AVOIDING/IGNORING** — when you are so angry you feel unable to speak calmly.
- **EVADING PROBLEMS AND ISSUES** — burying an angry head in the sand.
- **PROCRASTINATING** — intentionally putting off important tasks for less important ones.
- **OBSTRUCTING** — deliberately stalling or preventing an event or process of change.
- **FEAR OF COMPETITION** — avoiding situations where one party will be seen as better at something.
- **AMBIGUITY** — being cryptic, unclear, not fully engaging in conversations.
- **SULKING** — being silent, morose, sullen and resentful in order to get attention or sympathy.
- **CHRONIC LATENESS** — a way to put you in control over others and their expectations.

BANTER — A CULTURALLY ACCEPTED FORM OF PASSIVE-AGGRESSIVE BEHAVIOUR

I enjoy playful banter. This usually involves indirect digs or pokes towards another person at their expense. This quick-fire barb can build connection and be fun and it is usually enjoyed with friends or people you know well. There are unwritten rules in the game of banter and participants are usually aware of these.

However, the harsh end of the spectrum of banter can include abrasive insults, constant mocking and put-downs and be hurtful, exclusive and bullying. This is rooted in passive-aggressive anger expression. When this form of communication is the only thing that friends participate in, then people feel relationally limited and unsafe. Indeed, I have witnessed boys call each other 'stupid' and 'idiot' and men call each other 'wanker' and hurl abuse at each other. If this is the only form of communication available, it can be negative, hurtful and isolating.

4. Rage — Old anger

An instinctual rage outburst can be a primal reaction. If we feel threatened, we want to protect ourselves. We may feel that our life is under threat. There is no rational choice and this kind of 'near death experience', can result in a kind of protective rage which generates life-giving energy and power.

This kind of energy can fuel people in extremely dangerous situations, leading to extraordinary feats that help them to protect themselves or others. In a small way, I find myself tapping into this primal energy when I am on my road bike and a car passes me very closely at speed. In that present moment, my life rushes past me and I yell expletives and demonstrate with rude gestures, which appears to be a natural way for my body to release the internal energy. Expressing this primal energy at the right time and in the present moment appears to be healthy.

However, I think most expressions of rage I hear are unhealthy. This is a sign that old anger has not been processed and has become stuck in the body and psyche. It is an anger that has been unexpressed from the past. The past could mean ten hours, ten days, or ten years ago. Typically, rage has been locked in from anger experienced in childhood. Rage can lie dormant for many years, dwelling in the depths of our being, infecting our life and seeping out at various junctures.

Rage can infect our whole being. It can end up damaging others and ourselves. Rage can feel like 'opening a can of worms' or 'lifting the lid', it feels dangerous and most people would rather keep it boxed up, rather than risk losing control

The problem with ignoring or avoiding rage, is that it can only be contained for so long and eventually the dam breaks and the 'sucking up' strategy breaks down. 'Passives' are at particular risk of raging. Rage is a volcanic anger that erupts indiscriminately over an innocuous trigger or situation. If the root and reasons for rage are not expressed, it lays dormant like a cancer and eventually, it will unleash its destruction on the self and others. Hot or external rage does not respect those who refuse to deal with it and will expel itself when triggered. Cold or internal rage will eventually just eat away at the host.

There is a primal link between rage and toxic shame. Rage is embodied and a 'felt' sensation. It is often expressed non-verbally and rooted in the pre-verbal stage of life. Its very energy is connected to the core of existence. It is literally connected to the stuff of life. I have experienced this shame-rage in my own life. My first experience of expressing rage was not long after I got married. I cannot remember what triggered it, but I recall emoting what felt like a primal scream, some deep sound emerged from the depths vocalised in a high-pitched, otherworldly scream. My wife of only a few months was calm but clearly frightened. She must have been thinking, 'what the hell have I got myself into!'

Much later and on reflection, I began to realise that this was to do with toxic shame, the female connection and the safety that my wife provided enabled this shame to be emoted. This encounter had absolutely nothing to do with my wife. I was transferring the toxic shame that I felt in relation to my mother. This primal wound came from my mother and her own wounds. What I heard viscerally and verbally was: 'You are a mistake and you shouldn't even exist!' As a little boy, the message I heard was that I didn't matter. This had a powerful impact on me as I grew up.

The confusion of knowing that I exist but I don't always matter to others!

This powerful wound of shame has been at the root of much of my way of being and seeking to learn how to exist in this world. It has also been the source of developing many coping strategies which ultimately restricted me. As a boy, one of the key ways of managing a lack of attachment, affirmation and attention from my mother was to avoid her.

In reality, this meant I made some good friends and spent as much time as possible out of my house and in the homes of friends and in the company of their families. I was at my best friends' home most of my teenage years and loved the family rituals and atmosphere. I can even remember that my best friend's mum actually spoke about adoption to my mother at one point.

After the incident with my wife, I decided to go to therapy. Part of the process of dealing with the past was to go home and meet the parents of my boyhood best friend. It was lovely to be able to thank them for their care and the love they bestowed on me. I was so glad I did this, as it wasn't long after that that my 'adoptive mother' died. After going to see them, I went to see my mother. My rage erupted. I was in her presence but using my typical avoidance strategy of not fully engaging with her by hiding my head behind a newspaper.

My mother was once again speaking in a derogatory way, patronising or moaning about me in some way. I will always remember the moment when I suddenly erupted. I stood up, threw the paper to the ground and went up to her. Using expletives I shouted, letting her know I'd had enough. I told her I wasn't accepting this behaviour from her any more. I cannot be sure how long this went on for, but I think it was only a matter of thirty seconds.

Afterwards, my body was shaking and twitching. It was as if I'd just moved a historical, traumatic wound

---

Not long after this, I rang my wife. I cried. I was in shock. I wasn't sure what had just happened and if I had ruined my relationship with my mother. You might be wondering how my mother dealt with this outrage. She responded in the only way she was able to, by telling me off for swearing! Looking back now, her response was almost laughable but it was perfectly in tune with her wounded-ness and the state of our relationship. After this encounter, there has been no growth in our relationship. Our 'normal' relationship returned to how it was: functionally dysfunctional.

However, within me, this moment of rage generated growth. The significant change was that I laid down a marker and established a psychological boundary. This episode generated an internal movement and a psychological 'growing up' process, which meant I could finally leave home. I felt my mother no longer had any hold on me and I did not owe her anything. I no longer feared upsetting her and could now refuse to take responsibility for her emotions and psychological wounds.

THE RAGE MACHINE

Rage is cyclical. Once it erupts, the body creates a momentum in which the energy has to move to the end of its cycle. It's like you are tapping into an old power or trauma. Hurting or pushing the person is not enough and it's not really about the other, it is all about the primal shame and the outrage that the raging person is feeling.

Once rage has erupted, there is no empathy for the other. Even if the other is fearful, crying or distraught it makes no difference to the person in a rage. It is almost as if the enraged has been locked in, they are not fully present and they have been taken over by an inner monster. The reason for this is that it's got nothing to do with the present and everything to do with the past. It often has absolutely nothing to do with the person that it's aimed at in the present moment.

Rage is like popping a cork out of a bottle. Once it pops, nothing can contain the force of the flow as it spills out all over the place

---

When describing rage to a client, I will often use the example of Road Rage to explain what may be happening at a psychological level. I tell a typical story about a road rage encounter. A person is driving along when someone pulls out in front causing the driver to react quickly and apply the brakes. A first reaction may include shouting, verbal expletives and rude hand gestures.

The incident may then increase in severity with the offended driver behaving threateningly and dangerously by tailgating, overtaking or making more aggressive gestures and being verbally abusive. This incident could also be taken to another level, if the person who is experiencing rage overtakes and then unexpectedly brakes. This may result in a collision. The enraged driver may leave his car and attack the other driver or their car. In extreme cases, road rage has led to violence and even resulted in deaths.

Why is this happening? It is madness. There is no rational, cognitive component to this and therefore it is more than likely connected with an inner trauma from the past.

Rage has nothing to do with the present
It has everything to do with the past

Let us take a more detailed look at this. The driver became enraged because someone pulled out in front of him. There are two ways of looking at this incident; either the other driver did it on purpose or they made a mistake! The 'ragers' will, of course, believe the driver did it on purpose. In a millisecond, the enraged driver is transported back to their child state and an historic, emotional encounter. Old, emotional data may then appear in the person's mind. This might include 'You didn't see me', 'You didn't notice me', 'I don't matter' or 'Am I invisible?'

The present feeling is connected to an old incident of shame in which as a child all they could do was suck down these painful feelings. When the car overtakes or pulls out in front, it triggers these feelings. Enraged, the rager will now make sure that he is seen, noticed and respected, to make sure that he matters. It is a classic situation of pay-back for past hurts, but he is taking out his frustrations on an innocent individual. In the moment of rage, the perpetrator gets transported back to the original offending behaviour or emotional situation. Psychologically, he is blind to the present moment.

I'M NOT AN ANGRY MAN BUT...

I have worked with lots of men who have struggled with rage. They usually say to me 'I'm not an angry man' but every so often this rage just erupts and they have no idea why. Ninety-five percent of the rage incidents they report happen within their home and with their intimates, often the female partner. Many of these men arrive at my office having been told to sort out their anger or the relationship is over.

Don was one such client. He fitted the description I have mapped out above. During the first session, he told me his story. I imparted some psycho-educational information about anger and rage. In the second session, Don began to identify issues around anxiety and shame. After the third session, with no further rage incidents, he grew a great deal in his emotional fitness and has not had a rage incident since then. He now arranges a monthly emotional gym session to exercise his emotions.

Feelings are rational, but they do not start at A and finish at B or take a linear, single line route. Men tend to dwell in the rational and cognitive functions, it feels safe and controllable. Part of my work with men is to raise the awareness of the rationality of feelings. The more we understand them and become aware of them, the more sense they make and the more control we will ultimately have. Top emotional fitness is when a person can be aware of feeling evoked in the present moment and is able to make a choice to emote it on their own or to the other person in a way that is not abusive.

I explored the shame cycle and building shame resilience earlier in this book. The good news is that it is possible to heal the wounds of shame. I worked with an ex-footballer who was locked into a cycle of shame and as a result of this began to use alcohol destructively. After just a couple of sessions working on his hurt and his shame, he was able to start steady and sustainable growth. Now after six months and infrequent sessions, he has become shame resilient and is in control of his alcohol intake.

5. Assertiveness — healthy anger

From the outset, I have maintained that anger is a fine emotion. It is positive and needed. The four anger styles are distortions of healthy anger. They are unhealthy because they ultimately end up harming the self or others. Without inner work, rage will remain a destructive presence.

'No' is one of the most liberating words in the English language

---

The core of healthy anger is establishing physical and psychological boundaries in which one can express what is uncomfortable or unacceptable. It is essentially the art and ability of uttering one of the smallest and yet most powerful words in the English language: NO! Being able to express your truth and what you want, without verbally or physically attacking others or yourself is a good sign of emotional fitness.

Rereading the Aristotle quote at the beginning of the chapter is a good start. I often think that in today's culture, assertiveness is teaching other people how to treat us, hear us and respect us without disrespecting them.

I often tell the men I work with how assertiveness can prevent us moving into the shame cycle. Everyday events can fuel shame. I had just filled my car with fuel and proceeded to the attendant in order to pay. The attendant offered me no courtesy or respect, no eye contact, no please or thank you and virtually no acknowledgement of my presence. I left that encounter feeling shamed that I hadn't been seen, heard, or respected.

Something had just happened to me, but I was not aware enough to be able to label it. When I got back in the car, I shouted at my kids and my wife. If I had been able to be assertive in that moment, I would have been able to acknowledge what was happening. I may have also been able to be proactive and ask for some courtesy from the attendant who served me. In fact, making a non-attacking response is usually enough to protect your boundaries. This is an example of an everyday situation and if we don't catch the shame incidents, they hang around or are dumped onto undeserving others.

Being assertive is ultimately a win-win situation, in which both parties are treated with respect and can take responsibility for their feelings. Like any part of emotional fitness, being assertive takes practise and rehearsal. We know this, because after such an incident like the one above, we often replay the encounter and rehearse what we could have said. Replay and practise are key things to do to become more assertive. Working on assertiveness takes time. Below, I have outlined some tips in order to become more assertive.

1. **Emotional fitness is key.** It enables you to be aware of your feelings, checking in with yourself about what is happening for you in the moment. Being able to label your feelings and to name the right feeling at the right time is important in assertive practice.

2. **Using the word 'I' rather than 'You'** is a good place to start when making an assertive statement.

3. **Stock statements** — Knowing and practicing stock statements can also be really useful. The following are examples:
    - Thanks, but I'm not interested.
    - I'll think about it and get back to you.
    - I didn't appreciate what you did or your tone of voice.
    - I would like to be treated with respect.
    - I disagree with you.

ACTION

Now, check out and work on the toolbox below.

EMOTIONAL FITNESS TOOLBOX

1. Prevention of shame/rage response — If you feel misunderstood, instead of repeating yourself and perhaps increasing the volume, try asking your partner/listener to inform you of which bit of what you just said they did not understand.

2. Listen to your body and practise physical anger release such as running, hitting a pillow, splitting wood and working your body. This can be really effective when this kind of physical work is integrated with emotional awareness.

3. Keep an anger log — buy yourself a little notebook or create a log on your phone, which will raise your anger antenna. Record the time of day, trigger, person involved, body sensations, other feelings and the outcome.

4. Check out with your family and friends how they feel around your anger. This takes some guts and a non-defensive stance. Receiving direct feedback is a useful tool to increase healthy anger. Alongside this, explore any roots of anger connected to your family of origin.

5. Work out what could be your 'default' style of anger. Practise becoming more aware of your passive-aggressive anger and take responsibility for it.

KEY #7

MEN'S INTIMATE FEELINGS ARE OFTEN EXPRESSED THROUGH SEX

'Never be cool. Never try and be cool. Never worry what the cool people think. Head for the warm people. Life is warmth. You'll be cool when you're dead.'

—MATT HAIG[40]

Many men love sex. On the whole, they cannot get enough of it. They appear to always be ready and available should the opportunity arise. The strong lure of sex can often get men into trouble when they struggle to keep their penis in their pants. Men and couples often arrive at my practice due to a sexual indiscretion in which typically the male partner has had a sexual liaison or affair and relational trust is broken. Some men will seek to defend their actions, stating that their needs are not being met at home and yet will rarely talk to their partner about their sexual needs or frustrations.

Men sometimes expect sex to always be available from their partner with no discussion, almost as if it is the duty of the woman to lie back and think of England! In this chapter, I want to explore men's relationship with sex, the psychological connection around sexuality and how to develop intimacy.

Sex is a lovely and beautiful act. It is, of course, natural. It is a powerful connector to others

---

ARE MEN SLAVES TO SEX?

'I can't help it', 'It's my animal instinct', 'I have a need to be satisfied'.

Some men believe they can't live without sex. They feel they have to satisfy their needs almost as if they have no choice and can't stop this instinctual urge. I have heard men talk like this on several occasions. It troubles me, especially in relation to consent and sexual abuse. This kind of thinking might lead men to assume 'women are asking for it' when they dress in a certain way or even when a woman just smiles at them.

The male attitude of 'I must get my sexual gratification' implies men have no control over their sexual drive and therefore they do not need to take responsibility for their sexual actions. What happened for some men to believe this?

A man's sex drive can be so powerful he will do almost anything to get his needs met. This can generate a selfish, addictive tendency. I think this kind of thinking can lead to a dangerous road for men. It has the potential of ruining relationships. Some men are driven crazy by their sexual hunger and will go to extraordinary lengths to fulfil their needs. They may take great risks which could affect their relationships, jobs and lifestyle. When this happens, sexual demands have become excessive, addictive and out of control.

Many men pride themselves on maintaining control but they will throw rationality and emotional control out of the window when it comes to expression of anger and sexual desire. This lack of control can end up being destructive. Being sexual does not mean one has to forego values, emotional expression, morals and thinking capacity. The question that needs to be asked is what drives sexual need? Is it biology, gender conditioning or cultural socialisation?

THE SEX MARKET

Do gender conditioning and societal socialisation drive men's 'innate' desire for sex? Or is male hypersexuality the result of how western consumerism has commercialised sex? Has sex become a commodity in which women are often promoted as sexual objects and sex and sexuality are great marketing tools?

Titillation through sexualising bodies is hard to ignore in our culture. Semi-naked women and sexually tantalising women regularly adorn advertisements used to sell everything from cars to chocolate. Men are inundated with pictures of women and are invited to look at music videos, newspapers, advertising hoardings, lads' mags, movies and of course, pornography. Every so often, this sex-driven market collides with nature and raises a ridiculous cultural contradiction.

'Women feeding babies in public is disgusting!' but... when women appear semi-naked on an advertisement for beer, it does not raise an eyebrow!

BREAST IS BEST

Men (and sometimes women) will complain when a mother dares to breastfeed her infant in public. Shops and cafés provide a discrete corner for women to commit this 'distasteful and rebellious act' in private so as not to offend the public. The complainants appear to be ignorant that their shopping precincts and TVs are adorned with semi-naked breasts. It feels sometimes as though the sex market has copyrighted women's bodies and have purchased the rights to all breasts.

The sex market has convinced culture that breasts belong to men and not babies, breasts are for sex and not for feeding infants, breasts are for advertising and not for a free drink. I have actually heard men discourage their partner from breastfeeding as they don't want to share their breasts with a baby!

KEEP YOUR KNICKERS ON LOVE!

The lingerie industry is another driver for sexualisation. Sexual objectification reveals the pressure for women to be sexy and to take responsibility for turning men on. The industry is mainly about women wearing frilly, scant and often uncomfortable underwear that many women are told will 'turn their man on'.

Women are often expected to be dressed up — like presents to be opened up for sex or dressed like little girls, with frilly knickers to turn men on

---

BOTH CONCEPTS ARE A LITTLE WORRYING

This industry is big business. It is directed and generated by wealthy men. Both women and men are conditioned within this sexualised and pornified culture that this has become normal. The fashion industry and the toy industry are enticing children at a young age, to normalise sexualisation. When little girls are encouraged to dress in 'sexy' outfits and to wear make-up at just five years of age, then this is disturbing. When little girls are already thinking about body image and body enhancements, something is very wrong about the culture we have created.

Our culture teaches girls and women, their bodies and what they wear, should exude sex appeal. Men are taught image is everything. Of course, attraction is incredibly important in the mating ritual but we are individuals who are attracted by different things. We have turned sex, sexuality and attraction into a commodity. As a result, uniqueness, quirkiness, individuality and difference have become marginalised. The result is many women and men get stuck in a teenage loop of lust. Relational maturity and growth as a partnership have been forgotten. I wonder if this is one reason why many relationships fail.

Personally, I find myself caught up in this loop from time to time. I can be drawn into the commodification of sex. It is an incredibly difficult thing to move away from, when it is so embedded in our culture. Boys and men have it rammed down their throats and into their consciousness. It comes through the media, gaming, movies, YouTube, pornography, advertising and social media.

The age-old profession of prostitution and sex work is big business; it is even considered as part of the UK's GDP (it was included in the 2014 figures). Sex work has moved onto the online world. Finding a prostitute has become easier if you have access to the internet. The services prostitutes provide are usually for men, helping them to manage their sexual desires. With ever-increasing connections made through the internet, many more men have struggled to keep their liaisons secret and have found themselves mired in serious consequences.

PORNOGRAPHY AND THE PORNIFICATION OF A CULTURE

When I was a boy, pornography was very difficult to get hold of. It could only be located in magazines on the top shelf of the newsagents. But in today's culture, it is almost impossible to avoid. The world is literally saturated with it.

> Sexual objectification and porn is increasingly normalised and is now the acceptable norm in many cultures

Porn is big business and employs thousands of 'actors' who are paid for their kind of performance. Many of the actors are dehumanised and traumatised through this way of making money. Porn is performance. It reduces the body and sex to genitals and people to sex machines. Porn teaches that sex is devoid of intimacy, relationship and deeper connection. It is just about the act. It is often male-centric.

Porn has become endemic in our culture. It is having a serious impact on emotional and relational development. There are awful stories of how this pornified culture is impacting the minds and behaviour of children and young people, changing perceptions of the way one perceives sex, relationships and intimacy.

According to recent reports, boys who have been influenced by pornography are demanding girls send a picture of their body or perform a sexual act on them before they kiss or begin a relationship. This is a deeply disturbing situation. It diminishes the person. It makes it harder for boys to move away from thinking that sex equals intimacy.

The Tinder generation — 'Getting sex is too easy. You get bored. It takes all the pleasure out of playing and flirting; it is literally two glasses of wine then back home for sex. There is no emotion. It is lonely. You can't have a nice conversation after mechanical sex. It's just sex and go.'[41]

The rise of dating apps continues the trend of focusing on image and nudity. It is worrying. Recently, a fifteen-year-old female client told me she gets fifteen requests a day to send nude pictures. The pressure on young people is immense. Maintaining individual boundaries in a sexualised culture takes emotional maturity and courageous resistance.

SEX AS SPORT

'Did you score, mate?'

Some men use language around sex that presents it as a sport. Sex workers are referred to as being 'on the game'. Possible sexual partners could be talked about using language such as 'is she game for it!' Men talk about this game in terms of dares and bets as an aid to improve masculine status.

Sex as conquest and competition is a common masculine brag where he records strikes on the bedpost and mates are informed how he played his pickup game. Books have been written about 'players' and 'pickup artists', particularly by the writer mentioned earlier called Neil Strauss.

'The Sport' is a UK-based tabloid newspaper which generally includes two things; sport and nude (or semi-nude) pictures of women.

The language used around 'sex as a game' reduces women to objects, sexual conquests or a competition to win over

This kind of simple language is generally culturally acceptable. Many men do not think about it and yet it has reduced sex to a game and once again moved relationships away from intimacy.

You can begin to imagine how incredibly difficult it is for men within a sexualised culture, to move towards intimacy without sex. To begin to understand how intimacy has been reduced to sex perhaps we need to explore men's relationship with their bodies.

MEN'S RELATIONSHIP WITH THEIR BODIES

The body is the conduit for our emotions. Learning to listen to the movements and sensations of the body can help men to get in touch with their feelings. It is one way of increasing emotional fitness and reconnecting with the full spectrum of intimacy. However, most men tend to build their body to make it more rigid and impenetrable, creating an exterior that protects their inner fragility, warding off any possible attackers. This survival strategy can also diminish the expression of intimacy.

Many men have declared war on their bodies. This is not a conscious act, but it's often caused by gender conditioning and the man rules. Men typically punish their bodies by being 'hard' working, building them and disciplining them with the common refrain, 'No pain — no gain' ringing in their ears. Boys and men have learnt the body needs to be mastered, disciplined, contained, controlled and preferably rigid. Men often beat their body, work it hard in physical pursuits and sports and expect it to be pushed to extremes that may be one way of keeping the inner fears at bay.

These practices can become addictive. Relationships are put at risk and the body is under extreme strain. There is an element of self-harm about this. This way of using and abusing the body may be one way of men maintaining some element of emotional control. I have worked with many men who expect to be doing sport every evening and every weekend but don't consider how this may impact on their emotional wellbeing, relationships and developing intimacy.

Men build their bodies, beat their bodies and work their bodies. Few men listen to their bodies

---

I can remember phrases from my childhood: 'being hard' was a sought-after male attribute. This generally meant being a good enough fighter, never expressing pain or being able to do something very risky. Hardness is a male virtue.

The often heard mantra 'work hard — play hard' defines what men think they should become. No softness is allowed, playing is not about relaxing, it is about winning! Men are taught they should also be hard internally, showing no weakness or vulnerability, creating a defensive, rigid, impenetrable wall in the shape of their body to ward off any threats.

'Real' men are hard, rigid and impenetrable

Often men have learnt they should act like machines, separating away any emotional content. They tend to be clinical, rational and decisive in business. This often causes men to disconnect from their emotional world, leading to disassociation, emotional trauma and restriction. This can create a dualistic incongruent existence. It can lead to hardness, with an inability to develop intimacy, warmth and empathy.

I believe this separation is unnatural. It leads to internal splits and promotes a divorce between the personal and the professional. I have worked with many men who in several areas of their lives claim to be in control and yet, typically in two crucial areas, lose control. The first area we discussed in the previous chapter - anger and rage are typically used to disguise men's vulnerable feelings. The second area is sex which is used to express their intimate feelings.

HARDNESS HIDES MEN'S INNER FRAGILITY AND SOFTNESS

In a man's world, hard facts or the hard sciences are more important than soft data or people sciences. When something is hard, it can appear immovable, impervious, impenetrable, solid, true and interpreted as ultimately the most important thing to be considered and supposedly unaffected by emotional content. Likewise, the computer hard drive is robust, constant and big. Being 'hard-wired' conveys deeply rooted concepts or values which cannot easily be changed or manipulated and therefore can be ultimately trusted. Hard workers are more trusted than people who do not appear to be pulling their weight.

To look hard, feel hard and be hard is the unspoken desire with the internal expectation that hardness will be the man's protection and source of attractiveness. Alongside being hard, men have been told they should be 'cool' which conveys a sense of distance, self-reliance and dryness.

I often tell men that maybe what we should be striving for is becoming soft, warm and flexible.

Perhaps men could move from being big, hard, cool and rigid to being small, soft, warm and flexible

---

Men are often accused of being 'dry', which could be an internal defence against being accused of being 'wet'. Being 'wet' means being soft, tearful and weak. Men can, therefore, be starved of moistness, with their tear ducts actually drying up. Of course, being moist or crying is associated with women. Some moisture is, of course, acceptable within the 'hard' man's world. Sweat emitted from working hard is always acceptable and the moist sperm ejaculated through the phallic hardness of the penis is, of course, acceptable and enjoyable.

THE BODY PART DEMANDING A MAN'S ATTENTION

I have mentioned men struggle to listen to their body but there is one part of their anatomy they give special attention to and will be in constant touch with and it is the penis. Yes, we are, of course, back to focussing on the penis. Most men have a special relationship with this external appendage, which is an ever-present companion. It gives pleasure, is a great source of comfort, demands attention but is more complex when it comes to rules of obedience and control. Is the man or penis in control of actions, thoughts and self-esteem?

Perhaps some men fall in love with their penis, focusing on keeping its insatiable needs satisfied. It may even become their best friend. What are men looking for from their best friend? It could be many things but perhaps a mix of love, loyalty, respect, assurance, obedience, pleasure and presence.

A SPECIAL AND PERSONAL RELATIONSHIP

Why do men give their penis a pet name? Because they don't want to be bossed around by someone they don't know

In many respects, this old joke has some element of truth in it as historically men have named their penis with human names like Peter, Percy, Rupert, Dick, Fred, John-Thomas (traditionally a name given to stud bulls), Willy and Roger. Willy is a common name parents give the penis and indeed I did for my boys, almost as if it softens the embarrassment felt and makes it sound like another 'member' of the family. I wonder if parents are worried that when a child used the word 'penis' it will offend an adult's sensibilities.

Dick is a common term of abuse, often used to mock men when they have made a mistake. The origins of Dick as a name for the penis came from a shortened form of dickory dock — cockney rhyming slang for 'cock'.[42]

WHAT DO YOU CALL YOURS?

Whenever I draw an erect penis on the flip-chart in a workshop on men, sex and sexuality, I am nearly always greeted by a round of boyish giggling. Men quickly find themselves drawn back to their naughty inner boy. When I ask them to give a name to the penis, I usually end up with a long list of names.

In the box below, I've tried to divide them into categories. This says more about the traditional name connection with the penis. You will notice the majority of names are connected to traditional male associated interests, including wild and untameable animals, hardware, machines, tools and fighting implements.

1. **Appearance** — Old man, purple onion, bald-headed yogurt slinger, boner, Mr Happy.
2. **Machine** — Love pump, pleasure pump, cock rocket, joystick, love shaft, pink tractor.
3. **Weapon** — Sword, pike, lance, pistol, rifle, poll-axe, chopper, pork sword, piece, purple headed solider man.
4. **Tools** — Prick rod, tool, the machine, cock, pipe cleaner, chopper, dipstick, helmet, pole, knob.
5. **Meat** — Angus McWilly, Hampton Little John, sausage, meat thermometer, big Italian salami, hooded hotdog, pork sword.
6. **Animals** — Hissing Sid, trouser snake, beaver cleaver, energizer bunny, anaconda, baloney pony, one-eyed monster.
7. **Miscellaneous** — Lady boner, Tyson, Dicktator, Schlong, Whanger, Todger.

This long list of creative names for the penis raises a few questions, such as: What do these names indicate about the function and feelings associated with the penis? What do the names imply about a man's understanding of masculinity, sexuality, women, procreation and love?

HOW MUCH CONTROL DOES THE PENIS HAVE?

Many men have developed a special, personal and loving relationship with their penis. Some hold the belief that the penis has its own personality and intelligence, which they struggle to understand or control. This belief and lack of understanding has convinced them the penis has some control over them and the rest of their body.

'When the prick stands up, the brains get buried in the ground.'

— YIDDISH PROVERB

In personifying this unruly attachment, they have paradoxically distanced themselves from it. This has often created a schizophrenic, dualistic and complex relationship between man and penis. Sometimes, men have used this dissociation as a reason for not taking responsibility for the actions of the penis, leaving them to be led by the rise and fall of this unruly body member.

When an unhealthy narcissism around the penis reaches this stage, men may assume no control over their instincts and defend their actions by saying things like 'I couldn't stop myself', 'It's not my fault', or 'She was asking for it.'

THE ROOT OF MALE NARCISSISM

Typically, men are more narcissistic and generally more selfish than women. Healthy narcissism is important for emotional health — it helps to provide a sense of confidence and autonomy but this can get distorted. If unhealthy, narcissism will grow into a monstrous elevation of self-image as a form of protection. Narcissism grips people who have lacked healthy affirmation, attachment, respect and love. Often, they were deeply shamed by significant 'caregivers' in their childhood. They compensate for this 'lack of' by protecting their inner fragility through self-love.

The penis has become an emotional hub for men. Perhaps, some men have fallen in love with it as a way to compensate for a lack of self-esteem and a way of resisting shame. Narcissists have become blinded by their own beauty. This has acted as an emotional survival mechanism, leaving them with a deficit of empathy. Likewise, men who fall in love with their penis, putting its happiness above all else will lose penile awareness and empathy.

THE PENIS AS AN EMOTIONAL BAROMETER

Physically the penis is located in a central, external position and is hard to ignore and easy to handle, hold on to and fiddle with. Biologically and sexually it has a central function and for the vast majority of men it can consume much of their emotional energy and responses so much so many have joked the penis is where a man's brain is located. This is clearly not possible but I want to explore if, through gender conditioning, men's emotional intelligence has in some way relocated to the penis.

When a man is in touch with his body, he is more able to listen to the wisdom of the penis and its erectional language and emissions. He will have a greater ability to develop 'erection empathy'.

It is impossible to control something you do not understand

The motion of the penis leads men to respond in certain ways. It can correlate to feelings. Through the dampening down of the full spectrum of feelings and the dissociation of bodily sensation, their hard bodies and clenched fists become their first line of defence against emotional attack, while absorbing emotional hurt into the body.

The prime storage container can often be the penis, which becomes a kind of feeling barometer. Many men have lost touch with their vulnerable and intimate feelings like love, tenderness, warmth, fear, sadness and shame. The penis has therefore been left to contain and express these emotions. Many men are suffering from 'Penis hyperactive disorder' or PHD for short.

DEVELOPING PENIS EMOTIONAL FITNESS

With little emotional awareness or penile empathy, men will abandon any sense of control, rationality and willpower to obey their sexual demands. For many men, women become sexual objects and masculinity is reduced to conquests.

The movement of the penis has become the emotional hub. Developing penis emotional fitness and penis empathy can greatly increase the man's confidence, relationships, and self-esteem. For many men, the penis can be a source of shame but increasing penis empathy, it could be the most important emotional fitness tool they possess in helping to reconnect with the body, emotions and intimacy.

Part of penis emotional empathy is becoming aware of movements of the penis and learning to interpret its rise and fall, essentially we need to tap into what Herb Goldberg calls, 'The Wisdom of the penis'.[43] For instance, many fathers reduce contact with sons and daughters if they find themselves experiencing an erection when they are in physical proximity to their children. This can be disturbing and might lead them to becoming distanced from their children.

Feelings of shame about what is happening could also ensue. Knowing the rise and fall of the penis can be connected to pleasure, closeness and bed clothes, a phallus does not mean you want sex. It could just be a natural movement or a sign of intimacy. The very lack of closeness many men have endured can make closeness all the more exhilarating. The lack of understanding of the movements of the penis and reliance on this emotional barometer have seriously affected men's understanding and expression of intimacy.

WE NEED TO TALK ABOUT INTIMACY

Intimacy is seeing and hearing the other and accepting them for who they are. Intimacy is intimate because it is an exposing and vulnerable act. I recently saw intimacy written as 'In-to-me-u-see', which is a good way of looking at it. When we are genuinely intimate, we invite the other to see us, to really encounter who we are as if they can actually see inside of us. When we allow the person we are inviting to see us, we open ourselves up to the possibility of pain, hurt and rejection of our true selves. We risk exposing ourselves — intellectually, emotionally or physically.

Sometimes when I am delivering a workshop, I will invite the delegates to spend time meeting each other by looking into one another's eyes and saying, 'I see you'. This can be difficult for many participants. Sometimes, I suggest participants go one step further and invite them to hold eye contact with each other for one minute. This can be incredibly difficult for some people, as they feel exposed and seen. I have been doing this kind of activity in my men's group for many years and it can still be scary.

As a heterosexual male, I have actually spent longer looking into the eyes of men than I have with my wife! I have often felt intimacy is about being known and allowing oneself to know the other. I feel intimate when I feel safe enough for another to see me and they feel safe enough to allow me to see them — I find the energy in this encounter is electric, beautiful and incredibly intimate. Intimacy is clearly not just about sex!

Accepting the other as they are and not as you would like them to be, is a sign of intimacy. When we resist heaping expectations on them and stop seeking to mould them into our image, we make room for intimacy. When we accept the other, allow them to be who they are and are prepared to live with the difference, we are then inviting them to reveal their difference. David Schnarch in his book, 'Passionate Marriage' describes intimacy as an 'I Thou' experience.[44] It involves the inherent awareness that you are separate from your partner, with parts yet to be shared'. He believes to be intimate means being aware of your inner most self and welcoming this part. Intimacy cannot happen without individuation and differentiation, exposing and sharing our unique different self is being intimate.

In my counselling practice, I try to reflect this in my strapline 'To be who you are', which is part of an invitation to intimacy. I use the phrase 'intimate strangers' with some clients to describe what can sometimes happen within the counsellor/client relationship.

My clients feel seen and accepted. They reveal things to me which they have never uttered to another human being. They feel psychologically and sometimes physically held. It can feel like an emotional orgasm where some clients will leave my room feeling they have been heard. They say they feel fully alive and they are literally buzzing.

Psychotherapy can generate these intense feelings. This is why it is important for therapists to manage boundaries well and attend regular supervision in order to help them work through difficult and beautiful feelings.

Empathy can generate intimacy. Self-awareness and an ability to risk is key in seeking to experiment with intimacy. When we are intimate with another and the other sees us, hears us and accepts us, then it generates a moment of at-one-ment and togetherness while maintaining our difference. When intimacy is risked, there is a sense of being fully present with the other, being open to the other and a sense of feeling fully alive.

When intimacy is reduced to sex, relational capacity and personal growth is severely restricted. When one is able to develop intimacy then life becomes so much richer. Part of the reduction of intimacy in men connects to the loss of sensuality or being connected to the full range of their senses. This is a common problem in a world consumed by speed and image. The subtle abilities to see, hear, smell, touch, speak and feel are slowly being eroded. They are being replaced by white noise, image overload, overwhelming amounts of words, info-knowledge, a non-touch society and reduction in feeling. Our lifestyles are reducing our ability to be intimate.

'A fear of intimacy has held men in terrible isolation and loneliness, though this is rarely acknowledged.'

— VIC SEIDLER[45]

There are so many challenges making it hard for us to be intimate: busyness, stress, responsibilities for children, mental health issues and screen addiction are some of the more common ones. Other barriers include limited communication skills, including awareness and emotional fitness. I find when I give time to listen to my wife and allow her space to be, she thrives and I feel ever closer to her.

I actually find listening to be an expression of sexual intimacy. Shame, of course, leaves a large footprint on intimacy. When one struggles to accept oneself, it can be incredibly hard to expose this self to others. Many people will also play games on the surface of relationships, creating a dance of illusory intimacy.

I referred to the loss of intimacy due to the shame men have endured as boys and the way tenderness and sensuality have been modified so they are acceptable in traditional masculinity. By the time boys have become biological men, they have learnt this simple message:

INTIMACY = SEX

Many men have lost touch with their ability to express tenderness, warmth, affection, sensuality, non-sexual touch reducing their spectrum of intimate expression. When we teach boys to show no emotional needs, express no pain and suppress vulnerable emotions including sadness, anxiety and shame this clearly affects intimacy. How do men learn to express intimacy differently?

PERHAPS MEN ARE SUFFERING FROM AN INTIMACY DEFICIT

I published an article for professionals on men and intimacy hoping to generate discussion. I was disappointed as the few who commented did not mention the subject matter nor comment on masculinity and men's relationship to intimacy. This is a debate and discussion that needs to be had.

I have had several male clients who have struggled with sexual dysfunctional issues. One man has had numerous conquests — but feels lonely, dissatisfied, bored and unable to maintain a satisfying long-term relationship. Other young men I have met are unable to sustain an erection due to a difficult past relationship, embarrassing, or shaming sexual encounters and the 'Tinder generation' effect. This sexualisation of dating has reduced relationships to sex, generating further isolation and loneliness.

Both men and women struggle with stepping into intimacy, as it constantly asks us to move away from functionality into a place of exposure and vulnerability. It is hard work. Most of us will find numerous ways to avoid intimacy, including embracing the delusion of romance, porn/sex industry, busyness, technology and addictions. To be intimate involves an intentional way of being and that takes energy.

What are the roots of how men have broken off from intimacy? How did men lose touch with their softness, warmth, moistness and the most intimate parts of themselves? Many of the concepts in this book, including the trauma of emotional restriction and male conditioning, are part of this. The chronological location to intimacy reduction can be found in a certain time in male development and is what I have called the intimacy break.

THE INTIMACY BREAK

Puberty is a difficult period for all young people. During this stage of development, the young person's brain is literally being rewired. Their brains are flooded with a surge of chemicals, and their bodies begin to change in front of their eyes. If nothing else, this can be a confusing and bewildering time. Young people find themselves doing, thinking and feeling things that previously they had never considered. For boys during this stage, there is the added pressure of societal and peer messages, which strongly suggest what manliness requires.

One of the core challenges is the separation from the feminine or the mother. During the ancient rites of passage, boys were sometimes physically wrenched away from the nurturing mother in order to separate from feminine energy. This created a clear break between what the tribe understood as the differences between men and women. The separation is a little more subtle in many western cultures and yet, internally can remain quite brutal.

The intimacy break changes the boys' perception of the mother and female. Before this break, she was typically a loving, nurturing presence which generated emotional safety. During the break, this view of the female changes from the mother to the sex object.

The internet holds thousands of videos of women involved in sex. Female sexuality is used to advertise material things, with women acting seductively and as sexual objects. In the playground, boys typically begin to use sexualised banter, which often focuses on the boy's mother. How often is 'Your mum....' invoked. 'Your mum is 'fat', 'a whore', 'ugly', 'a great fuck', 'sexy', 'old' and so forth.

Boys sometimes share their attraction to a friend's mother, or more provocatively announce, 'I've fucked your Mum'. More cruel banter may include statements like, 'Your mum is a whore' and 'you are a mother fucker!' Of course, some sons can be sexually attracted to their mothers, which can be disturbing and, of course, changes their view and comfort around the mother.

Many boys can be left really confused about their relationship with their mother. Not long before she was just 'my lovely Mum', but now she has turned into a sex object. This causes the intimacy break. On one hand, boys seek to protect the honour of their mother and, on the other hand, they can't risk the shame of being seen as a soft mummy's boy or even as a mother fucker! They are almost forced into breaking that intimate, loving and nurturing connection with their mother to distance themselves from the female as a sex object.

This intimacy break may not be so profound if the boy has a male in his life who can demonstrate or model intimacy. Unfortunately, this is quite rare.

If men fail to address the intimacy break, they can often remain stuck on the sex = intimacy cycle. These men can become addicted to sex, porn and sexual liaisons. They constantly look for the 'sugar rush' of sex and are unable to develop more meaningful relationships. These men will have multiple relationships. They often appear to be 'trading in the older model for a younger version'.

They are allowing the phallus to be in control, with the aid of medication. These men are often lonely, stuck in the first half of life and struggling to grow up. When older men listen to their bodies and allow the testosterone surge to naturally reduce, they then have the opportunity to be free from the mania of the phallus and start to embrace intimacy.

'To possess a penis is to be chained to a madman.'

— SOPHOCLES

Not all women, of course, are naturally intimate. This can depend on their relationship with their mother and father. Some women may have learnt that sex equals intimacy or that sex leads to intimacy. Intimacy can lead to a fear of rejection. Many relationships remain functional, due to the difficulty of fostering intimacy and risking the threat of rejection.

For men to develop intimacy, they will need to consider the above conditioning, their understanding and view of women/mother and their unspoken expectations. To develop intimacy will take practise, overcoming the fear of rejection and seeking to embrace vulnerability. Below I have given a few tips in the toolbox to move from functionality to intimacy.

EMOTIONAL FITNESS TOOLBOX

1. Practise more non-sexual touching including hugs, strokes and massage. Once a day practise a 'hold on hug' — embrace your partner or friend for at least twenty seconds. Reflect on how it feels to be held.

2. Eye contact (soul gazing). Look into each other's eyes for thirty seconds, building to two minutes, without speaking and watch what happens. When you have sex, look in each other's eyes during sex and when you climax. (Note: this is not a staring competition!)

3. Notice moments of intimacy (in-to-me-u-see) in which you feel exposed and vulnerable and practise walking towards those moments, rather than away from them. Men — listen to your body. Practise becoming more sensitive to the movement, wisdom and language of the penis.

4. Men have generally learnt they should always be up for sex and ready to perform at any given time, even though they may not really want sex. Try experimenting with saying 'I don't want sex, I want intimacy' or if sex is available, saying 'No' and suggesting you would just like a cuddle, developing sensuality and warmth.

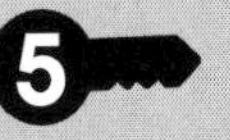

Practise reconnecting with your sensuality — tune out, turn off, introduce your taste buds to new tastes, do nothing, get into nature, listen and embrace silence. Practise the different forms of intimacy you feel uncomfortable with. They could be intellectual, emotional or sexual. Sharing your thoughts and opinions with another person can be risky and is intimate. It can be intimidating to start this process, but the rewards are significant.

KEY #8

MEN'S SELF-ESTEEM IS BASED ON PERFORMANCE

You are a human being not a human doing!

A client of mine called Susan told me she was unsure if her husband of twenty years actually loved her. He provided her with a lovely home, a lovely life and they had no financial worries. He was a successful businessman, but he was essentially married to his job. He worked long hours and was on the phone in his car all the way home. When he got home, he ran the bath and had a soak with his iPad and she might get to see him at around 9pm. He has never made her a cup of tea and very rarely arranges for them to go out. She is left bereft, lonely and uncertain about their relationship.

The above story is very common. I have heard it many times from both female and male clients. It usually features a man who is married and sometimes addicted to his job. He struggles to create boundaries around his work. He maintains that his job is to be the provider and he does not have the time or energy to do anything around the house, generate relationships with his children or care for his wife. Work has become central to his way of being. Why has this happened?

Self-esteem is a term that has entered our language relatively recently. It seeks to measure how good a person feels about themselves. Having good self-esteem or self-regard will generate emotional resilience and create available resources to be given to others.

Self-esteem can be increased by accepting and learning to trust ourselves. This is often developed by receiving positive feedback from parents and friends. If there is a deficit of this kind of positive feedback, then self-esteem will be massaged through other less healthy ways

---

Typically, men try to increase their performance in work, sport and sex, hoping it will reward them with external affirmation and plaudits. The problem with this kind of performance-based self-esteem is the storage containers are porous and constantly need re-filling. Men then find themselves competing for self-esteem boosters, trying to achieve more and more and in the end sport, sex and work eventually consume them. They have no time for anything else. At this point, addiction and a sense of being overwhelmed, can become the reality.

A reliance on performance-based self-esteem can be problematic for men, especially when their ability to perform is removed. When men fail at work, lose their jobs or become redundant, they often become emotionally depleted and can become depressed.

There is also a real connection with men losing confidence and emotional wellness when they become physically injured and are unable to continue with their sport. I have worked with several professional footballers whose emotional wellbeing is strongly impacted by being injured and side-lined. Injury is isolating. When men can no longer join in with their sport, they often feel they lose contact with their 'mates' and can quickly feel isolated. If you can't join in with the activity any more, contact is often lost. There is a male sense of camaraderie that comes from work or sport. When the activity stops, the friendship suffers as a result.

When the activity stops, the 'friendship' suffers

I loved football when I was growing up. I spent many years watching it and also enjoyed playing it. When I was in my thirties, I did not want to get injured, as I knew how important sport and exercise is for my health as well as having male contact. I moved to more non-contact sports and badminton became my regular activity.

For twelve years, I played regularly with a friend but I was finding myself becoming injured on a regular basis. Next, I took up cycling as my new sport and played badminton less frequently. This has affected my connection with my old friend. Yes, we still maintain contact but I now I may only see him six times a year. Our relationship is bigger than badminton but it has severely reduced our regular contact.

Men's drive to do and perform is driven by inner unmet needs and by a lack of receiving core emotional resources. Men often suffer from an emotional deficit. They don't feel accepted or approved of. They lack positive attention and secure attachments and often long to just be appreciated. Respect is often all they desire.

Carl Rogers explains how in person-centred terms self-esteem is nurtured. He describes it in terms of an internal and external locus of evaluation (LOE). If a person relies on their internal LOE, then their self-esteem will be nurtured from their inner resources and by trusting themselves. If a person relies on an external LOE, they will get their self-esteem boosted by other's affirmation. When an individual is reliant on an external LOE, the person could find themselves in a fragile state, constantly needing to prove themselves in order to get affirmation and boost their self-esteem.

Many men have learnt the only way they can get these needs met is to prove themselves through doing and performing. They have to get busy to achieve and perform to earn these longed-for rewards. They believe success, adulation, wealth and power will provide them with a deeper fulfilment.

Due to the male code and the trauma of emotional restriction, boys and men have not had the opportunity to foster their inner life or to practise expressing their feelings and thoughts as confidently as girls and women. As a result of this, part of their growth has been thwarted and they have had to resort to getting their needs met through 'doing' rather than 'being'. Boys and men connect through doing an activity, drinking, work or sport. This can regularly become obsessive and detrimental to relational growth and personal growth.

Why is 'doing' so important to men? We are not human doings we are human beings and yet somehow men have become a 'human doing' in which technique, performance and precision have become paramount. There may be a clue here in the old stereotypical patterns of men.

Traditionally, men have been expected to be the protector and provider, whilst women were usually seen as the nurturer, enhancing the space for 'being'. Men have traditionally been task-driven to fulfil the role of protector and provider.

THE MALE CODE AND SELF-RELIANCE

At the root of performance-based self-esteem is how society shows its approval, appreciation and acceptance of boys and men. Boys have generally been rewarded by how well they do — a condition of receiving approval and praise. How often do parents praise their children for their behaviour and achievements, rather than just for being who they are!

As a parent, I know I have not always taken time to tell my boys I love them and am proud of them for just being who they are. Boys and men generally receive a lack of approval, acceptance and appreciation, especially from their fathers. Doing something well is one way they can safely garner positive attention, within the male code. The male code rewards winners and often winning and competing has become so important to boys and men they will literally do anything to be and remain a winner.

Being a winner is all there is, there is no time for losers

The need to win — at all costs — has become part of the team sport culture. I often find myself struggling to watch professional football with the regular shirt pulling, diving and the so-called 'professional' foul. I struggle with the dissent, cheating, and lying. Some sportsmen will try and get away with anything and admit to nothing, as long as they win. This sends the wrong messages to young boys who watch the game and are influenced by their athletic heroes. This message can be learnt at a young age on the hard knocks of playground culture. Many boys and men can remember the shaming experience of being picked for team games. Being picked last from the line can knock self-esteem and when this continues repeatedly, a boy's self-esteem can plummet.

If they can't get their needs met by being who they are, men will quickly and unconsciously work out a survival plan which is based on looking after themselves. Self-reliance becomes their coping strategy and a way of seeking to get their needs met. Being successful and acquiring the trappings of wealth provides status, respect and internal and external power. Success is increasingly linked to economic wealth and material possessions and can be an emotional soother. Yet, the inner life is still 'lacking' and many men endure an inner trap and a feeling that belies their external confidence.

The coping skill of self-reliance ultimately generates distance between him and others. He has learnt asking for help is a sign of weakness. If he is dependent on another, he risks rejection and the associated emotional pain. Self-reliance has become a device of self-care but this protective strategy can end up driving a wedge between the man and his partner, children and friends. Men can sometimes eventually wake up to how their driven-ness has affected their relationships but often when it is too late. His children have grown up, his wife wants a divorce and he realises he has no friends.

Human relationships are not immune from performance-based self-esteem. Some men will want to attract a beautiful woman to increase their self-esteem. The whole pornography industry is based on sex as a mechanistic act and how men can increase their performance and become a 'sex god'.

THE HERO SCRIPT AND THE NEED TO PROVE YOUR MASCULINITY

A spin-off from performance-based self-esteem is the 'hero' script perpetuated and closely connected to the 'real' man script. The superhero comic scripts have mainly been based on men. These men are super and amazing with extraordinary powers. They are not ordinary men and they gain a lot of attention and applause for their superhuman feats.

Of course, most of us humble men will never reach such heights and yet the word 'hero' is often used for men who are applauded for perceived sacrificial feats. Typically, army personnel are called heroes, members of the fire brigade or the emergency/crisis services and other men who put their lives in the way of danger are also considered to be heroes.

Even good enough fathers can be called heroes, as being a good dad is often not regarded as a man's standard role. It is interesting how many men who care and look after their children are seen by women as amazing and called a 'great' father when this same care is naturally expected of mothers.

Fathers you are not a hero when you look after your children. When you spend time with YOUR children, you are not babysitting or providing a 'daddy day care' service. You are not helping your wife or partner out. When you spend precious time with your sons and daughters, you are simply and wonderfully being a good enough father

---

HOW DO MEN LEARN TO NURTURE THEIR SELF-ESTEEM FROM INTERNAL SOURCES?

At this stage in the book I am at risk of repetition, because one of the key ways of developing self-esteem is to reach inside and do the hard work of getting to know ourselves. The hard work of emotional fitness includes practise, rehearsal and forming good habits. This takes discipline and a regular exercise plan. The more we can get to know ourselves, accept ourselves, love and trust ourselves, the less reliant we will be on external affirmation, successes and achievements.

Nurturing self-regard is risky. One way of developing this area will be to ask for honest feedback from partners, children, friends and work colleagues. What do they think about you? What do they like and dislike about you? Listening and reflecting on feedback is really important, but we also don't have to accept it all as truth. Facing it can help us to develop inner awareness. One of the ways I have developed my self-esteem is by having therapy and testing my thoughts out in a non-judgmental environment. I have also been a member of a men's group, in which I can ask and receive feedback regularly.

Developing an affirmative culture at home, at work and with our friends is also a healthy way of developing self-regard. The British are not known for giving compliments or catching others being good. We know children thrive on praise but we as adults do as well. One of the best ways to get it is to give it. Start affirming your partner, children and work colleagues and watch what happens. It can be contagious.

Finally, it is important to foster self-compassion, to be kind to ourselves and let ourselves off the hook when we make a mistake or fail at something. Developing a growth mindset where failure is just part of growth enables us to become more resilient. Watch what you say to yourself and give yourself positive affirmations.

EMOTIONAL FITNESS TOOLBOX

1. Ask yourselves these questions: Who are you like when no one is looking? Do you really live up to the standards you expect from others?

2. Start to feed yourself by giving yourself positive feedback. Make this into a healthy habit and seek to prevent negative self-talk. Become more self-compassionate.

3. Practise looking for the best in others. Affirm and praise them, not for what they do or achieve but for who they are. Regularly practise using phrases like 'I love you', 'I appreciate you', 'Thank you for spending this time/moment with me', 'You are a beautiful person', 'I loved the way you responded in that situation' and other such thoughts.

4. Examine your work, sport, sex and relational life. Is it in balance? Think about what you get out of working/playing hard? How would it feel not to get these external rewards?

5. Ask for feedback from your partner, children, colleagues and friends. What do they appreciate about you and what do they find difficult about you?

KEY #9

ACTION IS A MAN'S TYPICAL COMMUNICATION STYLE

This emotional silence between men is making them seriously unwell. It is killing men, psychologically and physically.

Male to male communication can appear to be straightforward. It may include wrestling, touch and physical activities. Intimate communication could include grunting, a wink or a slight body movement and gesture and amazingly, other men seem to know the meaning of such discrete communication.

It is like boys and men have been socialised early on in their lives to the mysteries of the dark art of male communication. Nothing has ever been written down. It's just been 'grunted' and 'nodded' down the generations.

'Stop beating around the bush', 'get to the point' and 'stick to the facts'

How often have you heard the phrase 'a man of few words' to describe a man you know? Some men just prefer to use fewer words. They tell others to 'stop beating around the bush', 'get to the point' or just 'stick to the facts'. They might follow this up with 'If you can't say it in a few words, perhaps it's not worth saying'. Maybe men see words as a valuable commodity and refuse to waste them. On the other hand, perhaps some men just can't be bothered to listen attentively.

JUST GIVE ME THE NOD

Men can communicate with another man through a series of different types of nods, winks and eyebrow raising. It's almost like words just waste time. Body language is much faster! There is clearly something really positive when body language and gestures are recognised. But this causes real problems when communicating with women who have been more commonly socialised to verbalise and label feelings.

Some women think that many men have not really evolved from caveman style of communication with a full range of 'grunt' language and various degrees of nodding. In terms of 'nodding', I remember my youngest son giving me a nod. He lifted his head up to give me a nod, meaning 'hello', but then kept juddering his head back and forth for a series of nods.

It was almost like he was trying to make sense of this nodding language by saying 'hello' several times. Women overall find this simple language inadequate. They may find it incredibly frustrating if they want to talk properly about relational matters and the man responds with stunted conversation, grunts and shrugs. Some men can become increasingly mute if they feel threatened or struggle to engage and may eventually just leave the room. The woman is then often left to take responsibility for unexpressed feelings.

Meanwhile, the man may retreat to his cave, which could take the form of a shed, a location for sport, the pub, the garden, or some other self-comforting habits. In silence and often by himself, he will seek to allow the previous encounter to process through his internal emotional filter system.

This system, unfortunately, has never been upgraded and therefore it doesn't cope well with growth or learning. Usually, it just filters out the feeling content and the sentiment lies silently inside, steadily building up. He will then often emerge 'back to normal' and carry on, as if that encounter never happened.

THE SCHOOL OF BANTER

After body language, the next most common form of communication style between men is banter touched on in an earlier chapter. Most boys and men are schooled in this form of communication, from an early age. The basis of banter is about making contact with other men, through humour and usually at the other person's expense. It is often done in a competitive and combative manner.

On one level, banter is fun and can be an enjoyable way of being with others who like to partake in such communication. There is, however, a more destructive edge to banter, when it becomes a passive-aggressive way of communicating. This can be problematic in developing relationships.

At the extreme end of the spectrum, banter can get nasty — it turns into bullying. All kinds of unhealthy behaviour can be put under the 'banter' bracket: racism, sexism, homophobia and verbal abuse. Banter is indirect and inauthentic communication and eventually becomes tiresome. Often men will struggle to communicate with women because male banter is the only communication style they know. There can be a clash, due to a lack of direct communication and emotional language.

Men struggle to know what the woman wants, as they haven't been trained in other forms of communication. In terms of men coming from Mars and women travelling from Venus, I think it would be more accurate to say that men are schooled in banter and women are schooled in listening. In the school of banter, boys learn the unwritten rules of how to speak 'banterish', which includes the following rules:

THE SEVEN RULES OF BANTER

- Know the rules
- Be funny
- Be quick-witted
- Never respond with defensiveness
- Use banter appropriate to the stage of your relationship
- Leave it in the moment
- Stay in the game or be excluded from the group

Banter as a communication technique, when understood by both parties, can be a sign of a good and safe friendship. Banter can be interpreted as 'I like you' or 'You are okay' or 'I feel safe with you'. Calling a mate 'a wanker' can be a term of endearment and could be translated as 'I love you'.

WHY BANTER IS NOT ENOUGH

The difficulty for men whose communication skills begin and end with banter, is that it can leave relationships feeling stilted and stuck. Many men might be happy with the casual nature of banter and see no need for the relationship to develop. Some, however, may be silently hoping for greater depth and are fearful or unsure how to communicate in any other way.

I often tell the story about two men who have been best mates for twenty-five years and have spent nearly every weekend playing football, fishing or with their heads under a car bonnet. Their communication has never progressed from talking about the game, work, or women. They have never been able to tell each other how much their friendship means. Many men will not think there is a problem and yet a lack of more authentic communication leaves men lonely and emotionally isolated.

The toxic male cocktail
Shame + alexithymia + male code =
emotional isolation and self-destruction

As mentioned previously in this book, the male code and the trauma of emotional restriction is taking its toll on the emotional wellbeing of men. The toxic mixture of the cycle of shame and emotional muteness (alexithymia) is driving men to self-harm and may sometimes result in suicide.

Jonny, a male client of mine, described to me how his life had become a car crash. The survival techniques he had learnt from his dad and peers, were alcohol and sex. These, unsurprisingly, were no longer working. They were old coping strategies and were not dealing with the uncomfortable feelings of loneliness, isolation and failure. If left unaddressed, these difficult issues could emotionally and physically kill men.

Tom, another young client of mine, had been coming to see me about anxiety. On one particular session, he slumped down into the chair and with tears in his eyes, told me he was lonely. Until this session, he had been emotionally distant. He talked about his struggle with anxiety, which often presented in sweating. By talking about his loneliness and his truth, he cried and the sweat receded.

A big hindrance to move away from banter is that many men remain unsure if they can trust other men with their innermost secrets. Will his friend be able to listen to him about problems in his marriage? Can his friend sit with him in his pain? He may fear being accused of whinging and whining and told to man up. For men who are struggling with mental health issues, their emotional isolation can leave them fearful of sharing their struggles with their friends being anxious about how they could respond.

Men are committing suicide at an alarming rate. When a man kills himself, the reaction from friends and family is often one of disbelief. They are left shocked and may say something like, 'He seemed so happy' or 'He never said anything'. They had no idea what was going on inside the heart and mind of that person. Banter is not enough for men to develop close relationships with women, partners, friends, mates and children.

JUST TALKING ABOUT FOOTBALL, GAMES, TOOLS, WORK AND WOMEN IS NOT ENOUGH

When men are not engaging in banter, the next stage of communication is to connect with other men through stereotypical commonalities such as football, games, tools, cars, work and women. This kind of communication could be considered small talk, in which men talk about safe surface topics of conversation. Many men can happily spend many hours talking about these things, as the following story shows:

A husband and wife attended a party with friends and yet they came away from the event with completely different levels of information. The wife discovered their friends were struggling in their relationship, were attending therapy and having problems with their children. The husband discovered his mate had bought a new drill and heard the details of a new DIY project.

THE HIDDEN EXPECTATIONS IN RELATIONAL COMMUNICATION

'You're doing my head in' or 'you're messing with my head' are common expressions men use when they feel women do not understand what they are saying. Men commonly and proudly stay in their 'head', dwelling in the rational, cognitive and factual. When a man feels misunderstood, shame is often not far from the door. There is so much going on here for men in their relationships with women.

Many men have an expectation that women will magically know what is going on inside their heads. They think women will know what they are feeling, what they want and like, without the man ever having to articulate it. Women with their supernatural powers of intuition are expected to know all these things and are perhaps expected to ultimately take responsibility when communication breaks down.

This is also an example of how over-parenting can be unhelpful for children. Parents may end up feeling like in-house slaves. Of course, there are stages in childhood development, but to prepare boys for effective relational communication, they need to understand that their mum does not live inside their heads. This expectation can be multiplied when it relates to the emotional world of men. As we have already observed, men have a low spectrum of emotional connection and traditionally there has been a reliance on women to do the emotional and social engagement within the relationship.

Men learn during their boyhood that Mum is the person to go to if they are feeling upset or need to talk about their feelings. Men may translate this information into their adult relationships, as often their wives are the ones who deal with emotional issues in the relationship. When the man feels misunderstood, it's almost like his inner boy is left perplexed, hurt and shamed. He may then defend his vulnerable feelings by projecting these feelings onto her.

When a man is unengaged with his feelings and feels misunderstood, he might respond in various ways. He may take no responsibility or try to communicate differently, thinking it must be her fault or she didn't hear him properly. He may also become patronising — raising his voice and pronouncing the same words very slowly like an ignorant English tourist speaking loudly when he isn't understood. Accompanying this type of speech may also be a more aggressive tone.

DO...YOU...SPEAK...ENGLISH?

I expect this kind of communication from a child and I have heard this kind of language from my sons when they were younger. My son may start to talk about an issue without explaining the context and expect me to instantly know what he is referring to. When I don't understand straight away, he can get angry because he believes I should know what is going on in his head at all times.

I HAVE TO TAKE RESPONSIBILITY FOR WHAT AND HOW I COMMUNICATE.

When men feel misunderstood, they can often feel shame. This is why they ping back the shame through patronising or angry tones. I often show men a little trick to prevent the ping back. The first step is to take full responsibility for your own communication and in making yourself understood. Secondly, the man needs to learn to let go of the expectation that his wife, partner or friend will automatically understand what he is saying. Thirdly, try this trick: If the other person doesn't fully understand what you are saying, try responding with the following sentence, "Could you help me by telling me which part of what I said you didn't understand?"

This simple technique can give a little time to move from a reaction to a response. This can stop defensive and attacking behaviour and help prevent the man from feeling ashamed. It also helps the talker to understand what the listener is struggling to comprehend and prevents repetition of the same sentence.

GIFTS ARE NOT ENOUGH

'Diamonds are a girl's best friend!' is a cliché about the way women love expensive gifts. Giving gifts to our loved one is a lovely thing to do but it's not enough to nurture a fulfilling relationship. During the honeymoon period of a relationship, gifts, surprises and thoughtfulness come easier. However, when the relationship becomes more substantial or longer-term, two things begin to happen.

Firstly, like in many relationships, the gifts and surprises begin to dry up due to the busyness of life. Functionality takes over. Work needs to be done, the kids need picking up, there is ironing to do, etc. The gifts turn into doing practical things around the house. Sometimes, men can resent these jobs. They secretly expect to be thanked for helping out their wife around the house! Both men and women have been conditioned to think the home is the woman's responsibility. I have often felt surprised when my wife has thanked me for doing a job around the house, as if I was doing her a favour.

Secondly, the female tends to want more; they want to know what he feels, what is going on inside his head, to be conversed with intimately and to be listened to. Men remain untrained in the mysteries of emotional communication and this is often where problems in relationships begin. For contact and connection to grow in long-term relationships, the emotional connection cannot be ignored.

Men can sometimes feel confused when their partner complains about the lack of love and respond by saying 'I show you how much I love you by doing things.' Men can often say they will do 'anything to keep her happy'. When working with couples, one of the first myths I seek to dispel is that one of the roles of our partner is to make the other happy. One of my mantras as a psychotherapist is, 'no one can make another person feel anything'. My feelings are a response to a certain situation and may indeed be predictable, but this is certainly not guaranteed and is purely my choice.

'ANYTHING TO KEEP HER HAPPY' — WHEN SHE IS HAPPY, I AM HAPPY

This concept has its roots in the relationship between mother and son. Like in any family of origin, the unmet needs of one generation can manifest themselves in the expectations of the next. When a mother has unmet needs from her own father, this can manifest itself as a complaint towards her husband or her sons. She may have experienced her father being great at DIY, whereas her husband is not. As a result, she may think less of him as a 'real' man when compared with her own dad.

Equally, a son may pick up that Mum is unhappy. He may feel useless and uncomfortable with Mum being unhappy and may feel responsible to 'make' her feel happy again. Her son is also aware he may be blamed for her unhappiness and will seek to attend to her, as much as possible. The rule he learns very early on equates his Mother's happiness with how he is treated. 'When Mum is happy then she is happy with me and my needs will be met more fully as a result.' This is the lesson he will take into his adult relationship. The man thinks: 'If my wife is happy, life will be tolerable and she will more likely meet my needs.'

Often the rationale behind the 'keeping her happy' philosophy is, that if the female is happy, she will be happier with granting me more 'play' time or 'pass-outs' to be out with the lads and there could also be more opportunities for sex. This kind of thinking keeps the man in the boy part of himself.

If I can keep her happy then she will allow me more time to do what I want to do or be less 'on my back'

On the occasions when a man feels he is ticking all the boxes and yet still receives a complaint, this is when his frustration may show. This feeling may be quite intense and could be connected to the past. It might bring up feelings of failure, shame and memories of harsh words spoken to him when he was much younger, perhaps from his own mother.

This complaint can often send shudders down his spine as he has been working hard to avoid this. At this point, he has clearly been viewing his female partner as his mother and once again feels he has disappointed her.

COMMUNICATION IS COMPLEX

As a psychotherapist, I spend most of my time listening. Some people will say, 'what, you get paid to sit with someone and listen to them, surely anyone can do that?' Yes, many people can develop the skills but active listening is not easy, it is complex. If we were to observe our social interactions with others, there is very little listening going on. During some social occasions, conversations can include people actually speaking at the same time, just seeking to fill the space with some kind of noise. Let's face it, many of us are fearful of silence and fearful of really listening to ourselves, which can make it difficult to fully hear the other.

This kind of social interaction is filled with anxiety. We are desperate to hear the sound of our own voice, to make some kind of contribution to the encounter, to show we actually matter. The social encounter can actually be a very lonely experience, leaving us with a sense of despair and perhaps needing alcohol or some other substance to enable us to get through it. Many people find social interactions challenging. Sometimes, men would prefer to avoid them altogether.

Most communication is rooted in conversation which typically involves one person talking whilst the other is quiet. The person who is quiet can often be thinking about what they are going to say once the other stops talking. This may or may not be connected to what the other person is speaking about.

No communication happens without good listening

This kind of encounter happens frequently in every relationship. For example, when my wife and I return home from work, we tend to connect by talking about our day. Typically, my wife is generally better at talking in detail about her day than I am. When we both need to talk and require some attention we can fall into the above trap.

Men are often accused of being useless at listening. Typically, women talk more and men are expected to listen or at least be quiet. They may feign this with heads behind papers or smartphones. They may offer the occasional 'uh-huh' grunt of 'yeah', just to indicate they are able to multi-task and hopefully keep her happy. Typically, the frustration for many women is that when asked about their day, most men will respond by saying very little, giving no detail and offering no conversation. Women can feel a pressure to fill the space and are frustrated their male partner does not speak more.

Men may resent this but will often not try to change their own part in the equation. They will usually want to work out their day through some physical activity, sitting in front of a screen, time alone or drinking down the pub with their mates. Many men need to relearn how to talk about themselves but this can be full of risks. Talking is vulnerable due to the fear that the listener is unable to give you the attention you need.

When I talk to my wife, I want her undivided attention. I feel vulnerable and am vigilant about maintaining her attention. I am quick to detect any sense I may be boring her or that I am not important enough to her. Sometimes, if I register she is unable to give me her full attention, I will just stop speaking or suggest perhaps another time may be better for her. Whereas if I was inattentive to my wife, she can often just carry on talking.

In discussing this, we have wondered if I see my internal pearls as rare treasures that must be treated with utter respect. Perhaps this is connected to the lack of experience and practise many of us as men have had in talking about our feelings and ourselves. Women can often carry on talking due to experience telling them this is probably as good as it is going to get.

Relational communication is extremely complex and much dissatisfaction can be harboured in the dance around developing deeper and more meaningful relational encounters. Inner frustrations may seep out due to dissatisfying communication. One of the key aspects of successful relationships is that both parties feel they are been really heard and listened to effectively.

ACTIVE LISTENING AND THE MAGIC OF EMPATHY

To be an empathic listener is to stay in that person's world and to show interest in what they are saying, to seek to feel their feelings 'as if' they were your own. To listen in this way, can feel like 'magic' to the other person. Innumerable times, my clients have asked me about this magic potion I administer. They feel something wonderful and amazing has just happened to them, when in reality, all I have offered is focused, empathic listening.

When I listen to clients, I seek to stay in their world, to share their frame of reference, to hear their story and effectively encourage them to tell me more. I am trying to show them that they matter. I don't judge, I rarely ask questions and I don't advise. I aim to intentionally show my interest in them, their world, their story and their feelings. Empathic responses could also include reflecting back the feeling I am experiencing in relation to what they are saying.

A deeper, empathic reflection may include uttering a feeling that the other person may not be aware of yet, but could sound like 'for some reason, I'm feeling shame right now'. Alternatively, I may have a bodily sensation that may be connected with the speaker's feelings. In my own body, I will feel pain or perhaps become aware I have tears in my eyes. What I have described above is emotional-centred empathy.

ACTION CENTRED EMPATHY/FIX IT EMPATHY

The majority of men have not learnt the skills of emotional-centred empathy. Generally, women are more advanced in these skills and are more attuned and empathic to their own and other's feelings. The more natural kind of empathy men are attuned to is called 'action-centred' empathy or as I call it, 'fix-it empathy'.

When men have a difficult or uncomfortable feeling, they need to act on it by doing something to fix it

Men will often use physical exercise and external activity to manage difficult emotions. This includes sport, fighting, self-medication, physical work, gym and sex. Men (and of course, women) use external substances to fix the uncomfortable feelings which can possibly lead to addictive behaviour. Using substances helps the user to avoid or numb painful feelings. Removing emotions has positive benefits in the short term but is unhelpful in developing emotional fitness.

Being too quick to move or fix emotions delays the ability to gain understanding or awareness and to FEEL them, which ultimately allows them to stick. When one seeks to remove uncomfortable feelings (through substances), the reverse actually happens — the feelings become stuck, buried and grow out of all proportion.

Action centred empathy can lead to high-risk jobs

One result of an action-centred empathy is that men are often good in a crisis. Men tend to populate the emergency services, military and high-risk physical roles. Most people are able to act in a crisis when their survival instincts kick in, but due to a male emotional restriction, many men and boys can naturally have an advantage in a crisis. They are able to work 'beyond' their feelings and this allows them to get the job done.

A negative result from action-centred empathy is disconnection from their bodies. Managing and acting in a crisis will involve high adrenaline and if this is not discharged, then the body may remain in that stressed or traumatised state.

When men are out of touch with their feelings and manage them by containing or suppressing them in the body, this may result in 'post-traumatic stress disorder' (PTSD). Months or years after a certain trauma or episode, men may suddenly become aware they are struggling to 'stay in control' or even to function in the way they once did. This can be frightening. However, within the rationale of the emotional world, it makes perfect sense. If feelings are not dispersed at the right time and are stored up they may cause harm later on. It's always better for feelings to be expressed at the right time, to be let out.

HOW DOES ACTION-CENTRED EMPATHY AFFECT RELATIONSHIPS?

The male use of 'action-centred empathy' can result in relational frustration. The typical situation looks like this: The female describes a recent difficult situation to her male partner, which may be about a work colleague or an issue with a friend or family member. Typically, when a male hears this kind of story he will automatically adopt a familiar 'action' mode. He will almost instantly start thinking of a solution to the problem. He stops listening.

The woman may not have mentioned that she was looking for advice or a solution, but just to be heard. The man will often feel he needs to be useful, why else would she tell him about her problems! He ultimately wants to make it better for her; he wants to 'keep her happy'. He feels he needs to do something — the emphasis for the man, is on action.

What often occurs at this point is the man will feel the best way he can be helpful is to offer ways for her to fix the problem. What he fails to realise in this situation is that the woman feels frustrated with him adopting the parental role and effectively treating her like a child. She is quite capable of knowing what she needs to do. If she needs advice, she will ask for it. Good listening is all that is required.

When I explain emotional centred empathy to the couples I work with, the female can immediately acknowledge that this is exactly what she wants when she is talking about her problems, she is not looking for the other to offer a solution — she just wants to be heard

I work with many couples in therapy and there are often issues around their relational dialogue, in which they flip between parent-child states. This happens when one person may adopt an all-knowing/authoritative parental state on some issues and the other person takes or is treated as fallible, weak, small and a needy child. These positions change according to the situation and the issue.

For relationships to work well, both parties need to move regularly to an adult state. Treating each other as adults usually requires emotional-centred empathy. When men develop this type of empathy, they move away from the pressure of the Mr Fix-it state.

EMOTIONAL FITNESS TOOLBOX

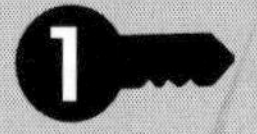

Ask questions.

A) When you feel misunderstood, ask for clarification.

B) Help me out — which part of my response did you not understand?

C) When you would like something from your partner, be explicit. Ask for it.

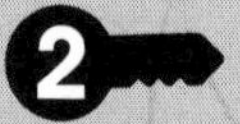

Practise empathy by seeking to become more aware of the people you are close to: your partner, your children, friends, colleagues etc.

- Look at their body language, facial gestures, hear their tone of voice.
- Try to work out what they are experiencing in the present moment.
- Try to enter their world.

Encourage men to talk more. Leave them space and try to not to fill the silences.

- Men — practise talking more to your partner.
- Try to move away from the normal topics of conversation and use less banter with friends and colleagues.

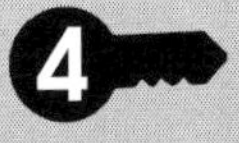

Practice this exercise. 9-minute exercise, building up to fifteen minutes.

- Find time in your week to sit with your partner.
- One person talks about feelings or about their day for 3 minutes and the other listens with full attention. If a person finds it difficult to talk for the given time, sit with the silence until the time is up. Then change.
- The final three minutes are for feedback.

Practice the art of listening in your daily life.

- Try not to be quick to offer advice or talk about your world, but stay in the other
- person's world.
- Use phrases like, 'Tell me more' and 'I'm really interested in what you are saying'.
- Reflect back what you've heard, just to check that you are hearing correctly.

KEY #10

MEN LONG TO BE IN THE COMPANY OF OTHER MEN

Leaving home and growing up emotionally is one of the most difficult things for men to do

'Billy no mates' is a common term used to shame men. Having lots of 'mates' or 'going out with the lads' is the way most men will keep this kind of shame from their door. To belong or look like you belong to a group and to prevent physical isolation, is an important part of shame prevention. Belonging to the male tribe gives a sense of security. Being part of the team gives a sense of unity, togetherness, community. It can bolster your sense of being a man.

Being part of a group of men and spending time with them is good for men. It is healthy for men to laugh together. Telling stories is a great way to connect. This also gives the possibility of sharing the occasional deeper moment. This sense of belonging is incredibly important.

The underlying message is that when I'm with the 'brotherhood' I am somebody, I belong and I matter. This is one of the reasons sport, gangs and teams are so important for many men. Being in contact is at the root of this, but many men settle for a surface contact and in the process may lose contact with themselves. Yet for many of the men I work with, their relationships with men are really about having company to remind them they are not alone.

Many of the 'mates' in their lives remain acquaintances; these are men that they 'do' things with and drink with They rarely talk about their internal and external struggles and joys with these 'mates'

This can often leave men feeling distant, empty, lonely and isolated. Quite commonly, it can also leave them with that awful sensation of feeling lonely in a crowd.

BEST MATES

One of the things I find annoying is when a salesperson speaks to me and calls me 'chap', 'fella', 'buddy', 'pal', or 'mate'. It feels over-familiar and pseudo-friendly. I normally feel mildly offended by this term of endearment. After all, I don't know the person who is speaking. On the occasions when I have asked salespeople not to use this terminology, they have always become defensive and sound offended, after all, they were just being friendly.

'Mate' is however common currency and how many men refer to their friends. Men will often greet each other with 'alright mate!' We have classmates, shipmates, roommates, soul mates, teammates and, of course, just 'mates'. The original meaning of mate derives from sharing and eating food or meat together. Mate is also commonly used to describe a spouse, co-breeder, and companion.

Personally, I have always felt uncomfortable with the term 'mate' and very rarely use it to describe my male friends. I enjoy male company and like being in groups of men, especially if we have some common connection. If I like another male, I would describe them as a friend. I think my general anxiety around the term stems from the fact that a 'mate' is somebody you hang around with and may even enjoy their company, but there is little 'knowing' of each other. Good friends and the men in my men's group are friends, they want to know me and allow me to know them.

STADIUMS FULL OF BOYS

Earlier in this book, I mentioned how difficult it is for men to grow up. It often seems like male development is stunted. Many men get stuck in a loop of continuing to do the things they did as boys. The lure of spending time with the lads, drinking and playing is so strong, familiar and comforting. These practices can cause an arrested development; boys struggle to leave their boyhood, almost like the prospect is way too scary.

Sometimes men's relationships can get stuck in the past. I have old boyhood friends who I have little contact with but still enjoy their company. But we don't talk about our internal world. The things we have in common are our joint memory of the past. It is often a relationship based on nostalgia. Some of my old friends have not physically moved from their 'village' of origin and have rarely moved psychologically. When we don't move physically our emotional muscles will not develop. If we continue the same practices we did as boys, there is a risk these comforts will limit growth.

There is a strong pull for many men to keep part of their herd or tribe. Sport often gives men this secure base, in which they feel safe in making contact. When a pack of men assemble to travel to a match, there is an instant camaraderie. There is banter, raucous laughter and joking.

Men travel in a great crowd towards the stadium, loving the culture that goes along with the scarves and team shirts, the songs, the smell of beer and hot dogs. It feels safe and warm.

When their team scores, the men are delirious, they cheer and sing and hug each other. There is a palpable sense of being part of the gang. In the football culture, with its rituals, language and symbols, men feel they belong. Watching sport, playing sport and being together in huge crowds can help them feel 'normal' and part of this common experience. It bolsters their image of masculinity and affirms their manhood.

I sometimes wonder if sport and sporting events have become a massive dummy (comforter) for the stadiums filled with men

---

These huge gatherings bring a sense of oneness, togetherness and belonging for men. As they sing, sway and shout with their tribe, this can almost feel like a spiritual experience. These stadiums, full of fathers and sons and mates, sanction passion, energy and express a much wider breadth of emotional expression. The sport relieves the sense of isolation for a brief period. The problem with the herd and tribal instinct is that it often limits growth and delays individuation, in which the person can express who they are and what they want.

BEING PART OF THE BAND

Men like to be in the company of other men. Unfortunately, this can also contribute to emotional immaturity. It is almost as if they fear that leaving their company will affect their masculinity and manhood. Do they fear losing their identity, their toughness and their way of staying in the club?

Men have to opt for either staying in the herd of boyhood or physical isolation. The bleak choice is between remaining a boy or being isolated and ceasing to exist

Many boys grow up joining clubs, teams, bands and tribes often based around sport, gaming, music and perhaps religion. When they are older, they create other forms of clubs. 'Old Boys Clubs' can include institutions such as the Masons or Golf Clubs, London Gentlemen's Clubs, Societies etc. Male members of these clubs and societies will fight for the right to stay separate and to exclude women, as they feel it can completely change the environment.

When men do leave the company of other men, the option is often aloneness and not having any friends. In working with hundreds of men, it is clear many men do not have any friends and feel lonely and isolated. It is difficult for many men to establish friendships in adulthood and hence the pull to stay with boyhood friends or boyhood hobbies. This may be the reason we find men in music bands formed in their college days and still playing together when they are in their sixties. What elderly women bands do you know of?

Men continue to play competitive sports into middle age and beyond because they enjoy the companionship and camaraderie, the banter, the contact and the connection. To be with other men in these ways reinforces their masculinity and their internal security. For many of these men, there is an internal fear of becoming soft and feminised if they spend all of their time with women.

THE TRANSITIONAL IMPACT OF FINDING A MATE AND SETTLING DOWN

Finding a mate, partner, or getting married can generate growth. Creating a new union and generating a new family is a massive transitional stage for many people, signifying a movement from childhood to adulthood. Leaving the physical and psychological safety of the 'family of origin' with the intent of starting a new family is a rite of passage, a generative transitional stage, signifying new beginnings.

In modern times, the state of boyhood is lengthened due to several issues including financial implications, longer life expectancy, lifestyle choices and expectations and the cult of youth. When I was a boy, the typical age men got married (the sign of leaving home) was between eighteen and twenty-five. Now, it is more likely boys will not contemplate this until their thirties, if indeed they can ever afford to leave home. These factors have generated a trend towards a prolonged adolescence.

When men get married or set up home with their partner, this transition can be difficult and full of challenges and complexities. The transition is complex due to each partner wanting to carry on their 'old life', whilst starting a new one. Expectations and new responsibilities can appear to be a hindrance and annoying, often causing arguments. This can be especially true for men who haven't had many responsibilities in their boyhood home and this can lead to relational conflict. With many of the couples I work with, I often hear the following unspoken expectations. The male will want to continue to work hard and play hard, keeping up with mates down the pub and partaking in his sports commitments.

Even after children have arrived, he may work hard during the week and then at weekends will expect to have a round of golf, go fishing or go out with his cycling club. This unspoken expectation is often non-negotiable, with no sense of this being open for discussion. His wife or partner will take one of two courses of action: she will just accept his devotion to activities and feel resentful, or she will risk questioning it and the inevitable tension that will follow.

WHAT IS THE DIFFERENCE BETWEEN A MAN AND A BOY?

I ask this question often to men and to women and I receive answers that include size, age, and strength. My definition is simple:

A man takes responsibility for his emotions, language, and behaviour

---

This has nothing to do with age and everything to do with attitude and maturity. My sense is there are many adult boys running around in society, struggling to grow up. In my practice, I have met men who are as old as seventy and they have still not grown up, they are still feeding and being led by their inner boy.

THE FATHER WOUND

The father wound is a psychological concept that Carl Jung described in his writing. It described a lack of fathering, not getting enough of father, not knowing father and the reluctance of the father to be present. I wonder if this is perhaps one of the core reasons men have this deep sense of loss, leaving them stuck in transition. It prevents them from evolving.

Not getting enough emotional presence from a father who is loving, warm and affectionate has left many men stuck in boy mode and seeking to be comforted by other boys. I have worked with hundreds of men and boys, 95% of them are affected by the father wound. Whether the man's father is alive, dead, unknown, emotionally disconnected but physically present — it doesn't matter, the father will continue to have a major impact on men's emotional health and growth.

My dad died at the age of seventy-four. I was thirty-five. My feeling was numbness toward him. I did not feel a biological or relational loss. I did not know him and he didn't know me. The sad thing was that at his funeral, I found out more about him than I had in the time he was alive. I felt cheated. I felt a great disappointment he was unable to give me anything of himself. What I discovered after his death helped me to understand his wounds and the trauma he may have felt. Unfortunately, he never felt able to take responsibility for his wounds. He dealt with them by 'going inside' with the wounds seeping out unintentionally.

I had a gaping and raw father wound. As a boy, teenager and young man I tried to heal this wound by looking for surrogate fathers and elders

---

When I found men who appeared to have more external energy than my dad, men who had an attractive personality, I felt a powerful sense of loss that I couldn't find an emotionally connected man, a father figure who could give me what I needed. I would become tearful, sometimes sobbing when I noticed a loving father-son relationship acted out in a movie, for example, some of the more tender moments in the film Billy Elliot. Watching the father learn to accept his son's difference, learning to embrace it and the caring moments they shared together. Even now when I watch it, I still cry.

I carried this pain with me for many years. It only started to dissipate when I began my therapeutic work and became a father myself. Slowly and painfully, I realised I needed to learn to re-parent or father myself. I had to find the father within. An important part of my healing regarding my father was attending a primal integration at the open centre weekend in London.

Two things stood out for me during this weekend. Firstly, half of the people were men. This is very unusual in therapeutic circles. Secondly, some of these men were at ease with each other when it came to non-sexual touch. My first thought was 'I want some of that tenderness and connection with men'. That weekend workshop was a very important part of my journey as it enabled me to do some powerful work on my relationship with my father.

There is a dearth of grown-up men in our society. There is a lack of tender, vulnerable, emotionally open, tactile men in our world. There appears to be few warm and empathic men in local communities. Ultimately, there is a lack of good fathering.

The wound does not go away. I expect to always have that emotional scar, but the impact of it will diminish over time. The way many men manage such wounds is to transmit the pain, pass it on, or project it onto another. The best way to deal with the wound is to allow it to transform us by allowing ourselves to feel the pain we have been trying to avoid.

DEVELOPING DEEPER AND MATURE FRIENDSHIPS WITH MEN

I began a community company called Men@work. The strapline for it is 'Helping men dig deeper'. The intention is to challenge the male code that prevents men developing real, deep and authentic relationships with other men. My sense is that for many men they have no experience of a different kind of relationship with other men, they have no idea what it would look like apart from a sexual encounter.

Many men will wander through life thinking this is as good as it gets. However, deep down I think that many men have a hunger for something a little different, they want more but it seems to hold so much risk. I want to show there is more, much more. The quote below from Gordon Clay is a beautiful description of what is possible. If you as a man want it, then you will have to fight for it.

'Man's inherent nature is to be curious, gentle, intimate, responsible, courageous, honest, vulnerable, affectionate, proud, spiritual, committed, wild, nurturing, peaceful, helpful, intense, compassionate, happy, and to fully and safely express all emotions. When will we stop training him to be otherwise?'

— GORDON CLAY[46]

MEN BEING INTIMATE WITH OTHER MEN

In an earlier chapter, I said that for many men intimacy equals sex. If this is true, then only homosexual men can be intimate with each other and there is no option for heterosexual men. The fear of intimacy usually prevents men from giving and receiving non-sexual affection touch and tenderness with other men.

Men have been taught it is dangerous to be sensual or intimate with other men, as it holds the risk of being seen as homosexual. Many boys have learnt they must expect to be distant from others, from themselves and from their emotions.

'Before most men can be intimate with others, they have to be intimate with themselves. They have to learn to feel and to be aware of their feelings.'[47]

There is no doubt that to be intimate will require men to become emotional and vulnerable. Becoming more intimate will not happen without risk, courage and suffering. It will also entail a letting go of the rules of the male code and the need for power. Terrance Real also guides us on this issue by saying 'When (men) speak of fearing intimacy, what they really mean is that they fear 'subjugation'. Being intimate is a vulnerable act that asks us to let go of being in control. It takes guts.'[48]

Intimacy requires passion. Men can be passionate about sports, sex and work, but can be passive about emotional and relational growth. They pass-on and demonstrate their energy for the things that turn them on. Passion ignites them and motivates them. The opposite is being passive, which is more about waiting, 'passing out' and being turned off. Men are often passive at home and in relationships, waiting for something to be done to them, thus men can end up appearing dry and boring.

The literal meaning of passion is 'to suffer'. Men are always willing to suffer to achieve success at work and often suffer in following their team. They will also be prepared to risk the suffering that comes with sexual liaisons. However, will they be able to accept suffering in beginning to feel? Once again, I draw on the wisdom of Bell Hooks when she says:

> *'To claim passion, men must embrace the pain; feel the suffering, moving through it to the world of pleasure that awaits. This is the heroic journey for men in our times. It is not a journey leading to conquest and domination, to disconnecting and cutting off life; it is a journey of reclamation where the bits and pieces of the self are found and put together again, made whole.'*[49]

As I have mentioned earlier, feeling our feelings is the biggest fear for men. But to grow, we must start this journey. I want to share with you one of the ways my passion for growth has generated more passion and intimacy in my life.

HOW TO FINALLY GROW UP — JOIN A MEN'S GROUP

> 'The group is somewhere I feel I belong, with other men, as a whole man. And a place where magic can and sometimes does happen.'
>
> — GROUP MEMBER

We need more men in society and fewer boys, but how can this be generated? Many influences in society seek to keep men as boys. One of the issues I find difficult in my son's lives is their constant reliance on screens and gaming. Their heroes on YouTube are young, wealthy men who have become famous for being funny and playing games. Many boys and men will spend hours being 'entertained' by this facile, humorous, and dumbed down commentary. Young boys no longer want to go to the moon, be a doctor or add anything to society. They just want to watch screens, play games and be rich and famous.

It is hard to grow up and hard for men to develop deep, knowing friendships with other men. When do men spend time with other men that does not involve sport, work, games or drinking? It is actually very rare. Even when men do connect away from the above points of contact, they can be accused of having a 'Bromance'. I hate this word. It appears to come from the male code handbook. Men being intimate with each other is uncomfortable for some in society and many feel better if it is mocked and ridiculed.

When I started the 'circle of men', a men's group I have now been part of for over fifteen years, some men and women thought it was a group just for gay men, almost suggesting that heterosexual men are not capable of evolving their relationships with other men.

The circle of men as a group seeks to directly work with emotions and work in a way in which they are managed without resorting to unhealthy anger expression. Typically, we seek to develop skills in talking and listening and guess what, men can talk, men can feel, men can regain touch with their feelings and learn to express them.

One of the main healing opportunities in men's groups is 'normalisation'— as soon as a man begins to talk about his internal world, all the other men are nodding away. The healing can be the realisation itself that they are not alone. If this is the only thing they got from the group, it's a real contribution to male growth.

WHAT HAPPENS IN A MEN'S GROUP?

A men's group is a simple space where men intentionally meet together, with the expressed purpose of developing emotional fitness and digging deeper into the inner life. We are expressing passion and commitment to put energy into meeting twice a month and we seek to grow and develop our emotional and relational skills. When we arrive, we greet each other with a hug and then settle down to do a check in. This consists of responding to two challenging questions.

1. How do you feel right now?
2. What do you want from the group tonight?

We seek to move away from a thinking state and expand our emotional competency. Men's emotional fitness is generally poor and often can inhabit just two states — normal and abnormal. Getting in touch with feelings can often be helped by listening to the body and is the reason why we do body work involving touch, movement, hugging and holding eye contact.

'The men's group is a unique experience for me. It helps me to understand and share my emotions and listen and feel the emotional state of other men.'

— GROUP MEMBER

The second question challenges the lesson that most men have been taught about self-reliance. We have learnt we shouldn't need anything from others and we should always be in control and never needy. The messages we have heard are 'do not ask for help' or 'do not risk being in a position of unknowing' as this could convey weakness and puts you in a disadvantageous position.

'A place where I can come to trust and be trusted by myself and other men.'

— GROUP MEMBER

The group may then involve helping men do their 'work' which means helping them explore or deal with a pressing issue. We may prepare a theme or do body work which involves movement or touch to help men move into an untouched part of themselves. This usually helps the group to work together. There may be conflict and challenge in the group which will help when authentic communication is present.

Below are some of the comments men have made about the men's group I have facilitated:

> *"Finally, I have a place to talk about deeper issues."*
>
> *"I've just been gripped all day."*
>
> *"Who needs reality TV, I'm buzzing! What a brilliant group of men."*
>
> *"I felt incredibly energized after last night."*
>
> *"I feel raw, totally alive and fully present."*
>
> *"I feel like a warrior, in touch with a raw edge."*

You will notice the aliveness, passion and energy expressed in these comments; there is no passiveness or hiding here. Men have been stretched and have made real contact being authentic, vulnerable and intimate. This group has been the place in which men have been challenged, accepted and have been real. It is a place that has also helped bring me out of myself.

When I established this group, I knew I wanted a deeper connection with men and the group is set up in a way that enables this to happen. I have to thank Bill Kauth, the father of Men's groups, who wrote the manual with a step by step guide to beginning a men's group. This book is called 'A Circle of Men: The Original Manual for Men's Support Groups'. This book is brilliant and in it, he expresses a credo of the group which encapsulates responsibility:

THE CREDO

- In our men's group, we each take responsibility for ourselves.
- To the greatest of our ability, we respond to our own needs and wants at every moment and trust that in doing so we will serve each other's greatest good.
- As I take responsibility for myself, I become a more real, authentic, and credible man for you to interact with.
- If I give feedback, I will take responsibility to tell you graciously about anything I experience that is in conflict with my needs or wants, trusting that we will enter into dialogue with open minds.[50]

Emotional work requires a response and we have to turn up for this work, there is no escape in group work, you will be seen when you are silent and you will be noticed when you physically move. The men's group demands a response from you and wakes us up from our passivity. This is why I need it.

At the end of the group, we check out by acknowledging what the group was like for us. It may have been difficult, fun, challenging or just boring; no one feels responsible for another man's experience as it is his responsibility to ask for his needs to get met. Our closing ritual is full of intimacy. We gather in a group, hugging each other and holding eye contact with each man in turn. If men want real friendships, they will have to take a few risky steps.

'The men's group is my community. It's a place where I can belong. I can be myself, warts and all, with people who care but are also challenging and real.'

— GROUP MEMBER

EMOTIONAL FITNESS TOOLBOX

1. Ask the questions: How many real friends do you/your partner have? How much time do you/does he spend with them? What do you do with them? Do you talk to them?
2. Reflect on this: When is the last time you went out for dinner with a male friend or on holiday with them?
3. If you have friends, seek to connect with them on a more intimate and emotional way — go deeper.
4. Seek to develop more friendships. Take some risks.
5. Join a men's group.

WHAT'S NEXT?

'You're a top bloke' were the last words Jack said to me as he left his final session. Jack was a plasterer and had come to see me about some relationship difficulties he was having with his partner. Jack was ready and wanted to change. He wanted to put effort into his relationship and into his personal development. He left having got what he needed.

The journey of growth and change is full of failure, hurt and disappointment with the occasional 'aha' moment that can propel us into new growth or a new phase of our life. You are the only one who can change you. Many men come to therapy when they have tried every tool in their toolbox. They then hit crisis and realise they can't help themselves anymore and need to ask for help. This is often an unusual place for men to inhabit, as they have usually been the one offering advice and tools for the job.

When men get to therapy they will often be in the child position wanting the expert or parental figure to help them and introduce them to new tools. Developing emotionally, however, is having the courage to close their old toolbox. This very act can leave a man feeling helpless, useless and can fill him with fear. Growth and change will come by him stepping into the unknown and beginning to move towards a place that for so long he has avoided. He has to choose to be willing to feel the difficult feelings rather than seeking to avoid or fix them.

Throughout this book, I have outlined how complex being a man is and how often our construction of masculinity has led to emotional restriction. Developing emotional fitness will take discipline and persistence but the rewards for men, their friendships, relationships and children are immense. I know that if men dare to feel and express their feelings, the rewards are great and they will have the chance of moving from a grey world into a multi-coloured cosmos.

Men can change and evolve. They can move from a life of emotional isolation. They can liberate their incarcerated feelings and dare to articulate and normalise them. When men share their feelings with other men, it is like a coming home experience.

The crucial step of change as outlined within this book is that men can change individually but to speed up this process, women and society will need to take the courageous step to change their expectations of masculinity and femininity. Challenging the prescribed gender boxes and our own formulated views garnered from our life experience is incredibly difficult.

Our expectations of gender have been burned into our psyche and just the notion of challenging those views can generate fear and defensiveness. I am under no illusion that the task of change is full of difficulties. However, if we dare to challenge our assumptions the rewards for individuals, relationships, men, women, children and society are great.

This book is designed to direct you to start this inner journey and dare you to share your secret life with others. If you take action, you WILL see change but I encourage you to use the 10 keys in taking positive action and in making changes in your own life. I'd love to see anything you're happy sharing if you connect with me on social media.

ACKNOWLEDGMENTS

My biggest thanks go to Sally, my friend, partner, lover and wife. She has been with me through the writing of this book and has been a great supporter, encourager, and editor. She is an amazing woman from whom I have learnt so much. Without her support, this book would not have been published. She read an early draft and then once the book had more shape, she worked tirelessly to make the book more readable. I love you.

I want to thank Richard Arkwright who was the first person to see an early draft, his brave critique was invaluable in giving the book a better structure. Miles Salter viewed a further draft and I want to thank him for his helpful input which inspired me to go back to the text once again to add whole new chapters to the final draft.

Thank you, Jan Palmer and Jane Masters, my two clinical supervisors for generously reading the manuscript and giving encouraging and useful feedback. Thank you for sitting with me and seeing me.

My final and professional editor is Kirsten Rees who has added so much to this book. Her generous advice and tireless work on the text has been invaluable in giving this book a much better shape and read. It would not be in print without her.

I couldn't have written this book without the hundreds of male clients I have had the privilege of working with and I thank them for trusting me and for their feedback. Working individually and in groups has been the greatest source for so much of this book. During the last ten years, I have tested much of this material out on the therapist workshop participants who have given invaluable feedback, advice and fresh thinking.

In terms of writing and exploring masculinity, I have to thank Jim Wild who stretched me and encouraged my writing and who first enabled me to be published. Thank you to David Jackson, who lives on my street and has been exploring and writing about masculinity for many years and has been a great encouragement and source of material. Thank you, Vic Blake for your wise work and helpful work on exploring masculinities.

I also have to acknowledge and pay homage to the many mentors I have had over the years, many I have never personally met, but have gleaned wisdom from their written work over many years. This book could not have been written without them and contains much of their wisdom. They include Terrance Real, Herb Goldberg, Bell Hooks, Sam Keen, Henri Nouwen, Thomas Merton, Brene Brown, James Hollis, John Rowan, William Pollack, Ron Levant, Richard Rohr, Bill Kauth, Victor Seidler, Lynne Segal, Ian M Harris, David J Tacey, Richard L Meth, Robert S Pasick, Carl Rogers, Will Courtney, Jed Diamond, Robert Bly, Susan Faludi and John Bradshaw.

I would like to acknowledge the male friendships I have fostered over the years that have informed me and being with me throughout this work. Thank you, Phil Frost for staying in contact knowing me more in many ways than others. Thank you to Wale Roberts for a man who I truly feel at home with. Thank you for sticking with me and loving me during our long friendship. Thank you, Duncan Dyason — you have always been an inspiration, encourager and consistent friend. Thank you, David Jones, for your friendship and support and fatherly presence.

I would like to thank all the men who I have shared men's group with and the men who have been part of my group and my life for the past fifteen years. Thank you George, Dan, Andi, and Richard for accepting me, challenging me and loving me. Thank you for holding me physically and emotionally. You are like brothers to me and reliable friends. I love you.

Finally, this book would not have been written without some cheerleaders. Thank you, David Sharp for being a great friend and an enthusiastic supporter of this project. When I have felt dejected and frustrated you have nudged me to keep going and also offered numerous wise advice. Thank you to Andy Paxton for your enthusiastic support, belief in the book, and for the whisky. Finally, my thanks goes to Rob Tucker for your regular book prods on our weekly dog walks.

Without the people I have named and the many unnamed, I could not have completed this book.

Thank you.

CONNECT WITH JAMES:

For public speaking, media, latest workshops, weekend intensives and retreats:

jameshawes.org

For therapy enquirers — men, women, couples, teenagers:

synergycounselling.com

synergyinfo@btinternet.com

@oneminuteman1

the secret lives of men

www.linkedin.com/in/james-r-hawes

REFERENCES

INTRODUCTION

1. Leonard Cohen, Anthem from the album, 'The Future', (Columbia Records, 1992)
2. Bell Hooks, The Will To Change, Men, masculinity and love (Washington Free Press, New York, 2004)
3. Albert Einstein

PART ONE: HAPPY EVER AFTER

4. Kyle Smith
5. http://www.pinkstinks.co.uk
6. Benjamin Lee, Printed in the Guardian (UK) Newspaper 12th June 2015

PART 2: THE MAKING OF BOYS AND MEN

7. Male and female brains work the same way; Journal Neurolmage, October 30th 2015
8. Vic Blake, Concept credited to Vic Blake

A BRIEF HISTORY OF MANKIND

9. Mark Simpson, Metrosexuality in your face (Printed in the Guardian (UK) newspaper - 13th August 2008)
10. Mark Simpson, The Metosexual is dead, long live the 'sponosexual'. (Printed in the Telegraph (UK) newspaper - 10th June 2014)
11. Dave Beasley, The Retrosexual Manuel — How to be a real man. (Prion, London, 2008)

THE RISE OF THE KIDULT

12. Joe Barnes (Editor), Are you a Gentrosexual? FHM Magazine - December 2013
13. World Health Organisation
14. Neil Postman, Amusing ourselves to death - Public discourse in the age of show business (Viking Penguin, UK, 1985)
15. Gary Cross, Men to boys- The Making of modern immaturity (Columbia University Press, New York, 2008) p240
16. Gary Cross, Men to boys - The Making of modern immaturity (Columbia University Press, New York, 2008) p248
17. A. Stibbe, Health and the social construction of masculinity in Men's Health Magazine in Men and Masculinities, Vol 7, No 1, July 2004, 31-51. London, Sage
18. Gary Cross, Men to boys- The Making of modern immaturity (Columbia University Press, New York, 2008) p82
19. Gary Cross, Men to boys- The Making of modern immaturity (Columbia University Press, New York, 2008) p92
20. Richard Rohr, Adam's Return —The Five promises of Male Initiation (Crossroad, Boston 2004) p32-33
21. Jeremy Clarkson cited by Efelftheriou-Smith — Printed in The Independent (UK) newspaper (June 2015)

THE MAN RULES

22. Dr Ronald Levant. Masculinity Reconstructed — Changing the rules of manhood — at work, in relationships and in family life. (Dutton, New York, 1995)

KEY #1 — FEELINGS ARE LIKE A FOREIGN LANGUAGE

23. Matt Haig — Twitter account

KEY #2 — MEN OFTEN FEEL THE NEED TO CONSTANTLY PROVE THEIR MASCULINITY

24. Joe Ehrmann
25. Terrance Real. I don't want to talk about it — Overcoming the secret legacy of male depression. (Scribner, New York, 1997)

KEY #3 — SHAME IS THE SILENT TERROR

26. Matt Haig — Twitter account
27. Karla Mclaren, The Language of emotions — what your feelings are trying to tell you.(Sounds True, Boulder 2010)
28. Karla Mclaren, The Language of emotions — what your feelings are trying to tell you.(Sounds True, Boulder 2010) p198
29. Karla Mclaren, The Language of emotions — what your feelings are trying to tell you.(Sounds True, Boulder 2010) p201
30. Brene Brown, I thought it was just me (but it isn't) — Telling the truth about perfectionism, inadequacy and power. (Gotham Books, New York 2008) p277
31. Brene Brown, I thought it was just me (but it isn't)- Telling the truth about perfectionism, inadequacy and power. (Gotham books, New York 2008) p280-281

32. Michael Obsatz, From shame based masculinity to holistic manhood. 2001-2018 anger resources. www.angerresources.com
33. Herb Goldberg, The New Male, 1979
34. Michael Obsatz, From shame based masculinity to holistic manhood. 2001-2018 anger resources. www.angerresources.com
35. Michael Obsatz, From shame based masculinity to holistic manhood. 2001-2018 anger resources. www.angerresources.com
36. Steven Krugman, Men's shame and trauma in therapy in New Psychotherapy for Men, eds William Pollack & Ronald Levant. (John Wiley & Sons, Inc, New York 1998)
37. Karla Mclaren. The Language of emotions — what your feelings are trying to tell you. (Sounds True, Boulder 2010) p207

KEY #5 — HE LONGS TO BE LOOKED AFTER AND SO DOES SHE

38. Neil Strauss, The Truth — an uncomfortable book about relationships (Harper Collins, 2015) p377

KEY #6 — MEN'S VULNERABLE FEELINGS ARE EXPRESSED THROUGH ANGER

39. Aristotle

KEY #7 — MEN'S INTIMATE FEELINGS ARE OFTEN EXPRESSED THROUGH SEX

40. Matt Haig
41. Lucy Holden. Broke, tired and bored of Tinder — why millennials are turned off sex. The Times magazine (December 1st, 2018)

42. Tom Hickman. God's Doodle — The life and times of the penis. (Square Peg, London, 2012)
43. Herb Goldberg. The Hazards of being male, surviving the myth of masculine privilege. (Sanford J. Greenburger Ass, Inc, Chicago, 1976)
44. David Schnarch, Passionate Marriage. (Norton, New York, 2009)
45. Victor J Seidler, Rediscovering masculinity — Reason, language and Sexuality. (Routledge, London, 1998) p162

KEY #10 — HE LONGS TO BE IN THE COMPANY OF OTHER MEN

46. Gordon Clay. Quote discovered on a defunct website
47. Terrance Real. Cited in Bell Hooks, The will to change — Men, masculinity and love (Washington Free Press, New York, 2004) p146
48. Terrance Real — As above
49. Bell Hooks, The Will To Change, Men, masculinity and love (Washington Free Press, New York, 2004) p181
50. Bill Kauth. A Circle of Men — The original manual for men's support groups. (St Martins Press, New York, 1992) p24